Pediatric Primary Care Nurse Practitioner Exam Part 1 of 2

SECRETS

Study Guide
Your Key to Exam Success

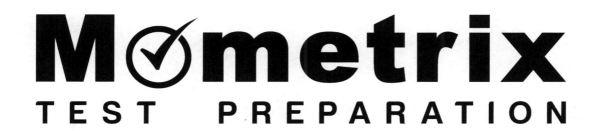

Dear Future Exam Success Story:

First of all, **THANK YOU** for purchasing Mometrix study materials!

Second, congratulations! You are one of the few determined test-takers who are committed to doing whatever it takes to excel on your exam. **You have come to the right place.** We developed these study materials with one goal in mind: to deliver you the information you need in a format that's concise and easy to use.

In addition to optimizing your guide for the content of the test, we've outlined our recommended steps for breaking down the preparation process into small, attainable goals so you can make sure you stay on track.

We've also analyzed the entire test-taking process, identifying the most common pitfalls and showing how you can overcome them and be ready for any curveball the test throws you.

Standardized testing is one of the biggest obstacles on your road to success, which only increases the importance of doing well in the high-pressure, high-stakes environment of test day. Your results on this test could have a significant impact on your future, and this guide provides the information and practical advice to help you achieve your full potential on test day.

Your success is our success

We would love to hear from you! If you would like to share the story of your exam success or if you have any questions or comments in regard to our products, please contact us at **800-673-8175** or **support@mometrix.com**.

Thanks again for your business and we wish you continued success!

Sincerely,
The Mometrix Test Preparation Team

Need more help? Check out our flashcards at: http://mometrixflashcards.com/NP

TABLE OF CONTENTS

Introduction

Thank you for purchasing this resource! You have made the choice to prepare yourself for a test that could have a huge impact on your future, and this guide is designed to help you be fully ready for test day. Obviously, it's important to have a solid understanding of the test material, but you also need to be prepared for the unique environment and stressors of the test, so that you can perform to the best of your abilities.

For this purpose, the first section that appears in this guide is the **Secret Keys**. We've devoted countless hours to meticulously researching what works and what doesn't, and we've boiled down our findings to the five most impactful steps you can take to improve your performance on the test. We start at the beginning with study planning and move through the preparation process, all the way to the testing strategies that will help you get the most out of what you know when you're finally sitting in front of the test.

We recommend that you start preparing for your test as far in advance as possible. However, if you've bought this guide as a last-minute study resource and only have a few days before your test, we recommend that you skip over the first two Secret Keys since they address a long-term study plan.

If you struggle with **test anxiety**, we strongly encourage you to check out our recommendations for how you can overcome it. Test anxiety is a formidable foe, but it can be beaten, and we want to make sure you have the tools you need to defeat it.

Secret Key #1 – Plan Big, Study Small

There's a lot riding on your performance. If you want to ace this test, you're going to need to keep your skills sharp and the material fresh in your mind. You need a plan that lets you review everything you need to know while still fitting in your schedule. We'll break this strategy down into three categories.

Information Organization

Start with the information you already have: the official test outline. From this, you can make a complete list of all the concepts you need to cover before the test. Organize these concepts into groups that can be studied together, and create a list of any related vocabulary you need to learn so you can brush up on any difficult terms. You'll want to keep this vocabulary list handy once you actually start studying since you may need to add to it along the way.

Time Management

Once you have your set of study concepts, decide how to spread them out over the time you have left before the test. Break your study plan into small, clear goals so you have a manageable task for each day and know exactly what you're doing. Then just focus on one small step at a time. When you manage your time this way, you don't need to spend hours at a time studying. Studying a small block of content for a short period each day helps you retain information better and avoid stressing over how much you have left to do. You can relax knowing that you have a plan to cover everything in time. In order for this strategy to be effective though, you have to start studying early and stick to your schedule. Avoid the exhaustion and futility that comes from last-minute cramming!

Study Environment

The environment you study in has a big impact on your learning. Studying in a coffee shop, while probably more enjoyable, is not likely to be as fruitful as studying in a quiet room. It's important to keep distractions to a minimum. You're only planning to study for a short block of time, so make the most of it. Don't pause to check your phone or get up to find a snack. It's also important to **avoid multitasking**. Research has consistently shown that multitasking will make your studying dramatically less effective. Your study area should also be comfortable and well-lit so you don't have the distraction of straining your eyes or sitting on an uncomfortable chair.

The time of day you study is also important. You want to be rested and alert. Don't wait until just before bedtime. Study when you'll be most likely to comprehend and remember. Even better, if you know what time of day your test will be, set that time aside for study. That way your brain will be used to working on that subject at that specific time and you'll have a better chance of recalling information.

Finally, it can be helpful to team up with others who are studying for the same test. Your actual studying should be done in as isolated an environment as possible, but the work of organizing the information and setting up the study plan can be divided up. In between study sessions, you can discuss with your teammates the concepts that you're all studying and quiz each other on the details. Just be sure that your teammates are as serious about the test as you are. If you find that your study time is being replaced with social time, you might need to find a new team.

Secret Key #2 – Make Your Studying Count

You're devoting a lot of time and effort to preparing for this test, so you want to be absolutely certain it will pay off. This means doing more than just reading the content and hoping you can remember it on test day. It's important to make every minute of study count. There are two main areas you can focus on to make your studying count:

Retention

It doesn't matter how much time you study if you can't remember the material. You need to make sure you are retaining the concepts. To check your retention of the information you're learning, try recalling it at later times with minimal prompting. Try carrying around flashcards and glance at one or two from time to time or ask a friend who's also studying for the test to quiz you.

To enhance your retention, look for ways to put the information into practice so that you can apply it rather than simply recalling it. If you're using the information in practical ways, it will be much easier to remember. Similarly, it helps to solidify a concept in your mind if you're not only reading it to yourself but also explaining it to someone else. Ask a friend to let you teach them about a concept you're a little shaky on (or speak aloud to an imaginary audience if necessary). As you try to summarize, define, give examples, and answer your friend's questions, you'll understand the concepts better and they will stay with you longer. Finally, step back for a big picture view and ask yourself how each piece of information fits with the whole subject. When you link the different concepts together and see them working together as a whole, it's easier to remember the individual components.

Finally, practice showing your work on any multi-step problems, even if you're just studying. Writing out each step you take to solve a problem will help solidify the process in your mind, and you'll be more likely to remember it during the test.

Modality

Modality simply refers to the means or method by which you study. Choosing a study modality that fits your own individual learning style is crucial. No two people learn best in exactly the same way, so it's important to know your strengths and use them to your advantage.

For example, if you learn best by visualization, focus on visualizing a concept in your mind and draw an image or a diagram. Try color-coding your notes, illustrating them, or creating symbols that will trigger your mind to recall a learned concept. If you learn best by hearing or discussing information, find a study partner who learns the same way or read aloud to yourself. Think about how to put the information in your own words. Imagine that you are giving a lecture on the topic and record yourself so you can listen to it later.

For any learning style, flashcards can be helpful. Organize the information so you can take advantage of spare moments to review. Underline key words or phrases. Use different colors for different categories. Mnemonic devices (such as creating a short list in which every item starts with the same letter) can also help with retention. Find what works best for you and use it to store the information in your mind most effectively and easily.

Secret Key #3 – Practice the Right Way

Your success on test day depends not only on how many hours you put into preparing, but also on whether you prepared the right way. It's good to check along the way to see if your studying is paying off. One of the most effective ways to do this is by taking practice tests to evaluate your progress. Practice tests are useful because they show exactly where you need to improve. Every time you take a practice test, pay special attention to these three groups of questions:

- The questions you got wrong
- The questions you had to guess on, even if you guessed right
- The questions you found difficult or slow to work through

This will show you exactly what your weak areas are, and where you need to devote more study time. Ask yourself why each of these questions gave you trouble. Was it because you didn't understand the material? Was it because you didn't remember the vocabulary? Do you need more repetitions on this type of question to build speed and confidence? Dig into those questions and figure out how you can strengthen your weak areas as you go back to review the material.

Additionally, many practice tests have a section explaining the answer choices. It can be tempting to read the explanation and think that you now have a good understanding of the concept. However, an explanation likely only covers part of the question's broader context. Even if the explanation makes sense, **go back and investigate** every concept related to the question until you're positive you have a thorough understanding.

As you go along, keep in mind that the practice test is just that: practice. Memorizing these questions and answers will not be very helpful on the actual test because it is unlikely to have any of the same exact questions. If you only know the right answers to the sample questions, you won't be prepared for the real thing. **Study the concepts** until you understand them fully, and then you'll be able to answer any question that shows up on the test.

It's important to wait on the practice tests until you're ready. If you take a test on your first day of study, you may be overwhelmed by the amount of material covered and how much you need to learn. Work up to it gradually.

On test day, you'll need to be prepared for answering questions, managing your time, and using the test-taking strategies you've learned. It's a lot to balance, like a mental marathon that will have a big impact on your future. Like training for a marathon, you'll need to start slowly and work your way up. When test day arrives, you'll be ready.

Start with the strategies you've read in the first two Secret Keys—plan your course and study in the way that works best for you. If you have time, consider using multiple study resources to get different approaches to the same concepts. It can be helpful to see difficult concepts from more than one angle. Then find a good source for practice tests. Many times, the test website will suggest potential study resources or provide sample tests.

4

Practice Test Strategy

If you're able to find at least three practice tests, we recommend this strategy:

Untimed and Open-Book Practice

Take the first test with no time constraints and with your notes and study guide handy. Take your time and focus on applying the strategies you've learned.

Timed and Open-Book Practice

Take the second practice test open-book as well, but set a timer and practice pacing yourself to finish in time.

Timed and Closed-Book Practice

Take any other practice tests as if it were test day. Set a timer and put away your study materials. Sit at a table or desk in a quiet room, imagine yourself at the testing center, and answer questions as quickly and accurately as possible.

Keep repeating timed and closed-book tests on a regular basis until you run out of practice tests or it's time for the actual test. Your mind will be ready for the schedule and stress of test day, and you'll be able to focus on recalling the material you've learned.

Secret Key #4 – Pace Yourself

Once you're fully prepared for the material on the test, your biggest challenge on test day will be managing your time. Just knowing that the clock is ticking can make you panic even if you have plenty of time left. Work on pacing yourself so you can build confidence against the time constraints of the exam. Pacing is a difficult skill to master, especially in a high-pressure environment, so **practice is vital**.

Set time expectations for your pace based on how much time is available. For example, if a section has 60 questions and the time limit is 30 minutes, you know you have to average 30 seconds or less per question in order to answer them all. Although 30 seconds is the hard limit, set 25 seconds per question as your goal, so you reserve extra time to spend on harder questions. When you budget extra time for the harder questions, you no longer have any reason to stress when those questions take longer to answer.

Don't let this time expectation distract you from working through the test at a calm, steady pace, but keep it in mind so you don't spend too much time on any one question. Recognize that taking extra time on one question you don't understand may keep you from answering two that you do understand later in the test. If your time limit for a question is up and you're still not sure of the answer, mark it and move on, and come back to it later if the time and the test format allow. If the testing format doesn't allow you to return to earlier questions, just make an educated guess; then put it out of your mind and move on.

On the easier questions, be careful not to rush. It may seem wise to hurry through them so you have more time for the challenging ones, but it's not worth missing one if you know the concept and just didn't take the time to read the question fully. Work efficiently but make sure you understand the question and have looked at all of the answer choices, since more than one may seem right at first.

Even if you're paying attention to the time, you may find yourself a little behind at some point. You should speed up to get back on track, but do so wisely. Don't panic; just take a few seconds less on each question until you're caught up. Don't guess without thinking, but do look through the answer choices and eliminate any you know are wrong. If you can get down to two choices, it is often worthwhile to guess from those. Once you've chosen an answer, move on and don't dwell on any that you skipped or had to hurry through. If a question was taking too long, chances are it was one of the harder ones, so you weren't as likely to get it right anyway.

On the other hand, if you find yourself getting ahead of schedule, it may be beneficial to slow down a little. The more quickly you work, the more likely you are to make a careless mistake that will affect your score. You've budgeted time for each question, so don't be afraid to spend that time. Practice an efficient but careful pace to get the most out of the time you have.

6

Secret Key #5 – Have a Plan for Guessing

When you're taking the test, you may find yourself stuck on a question. Some of the answer choices seem better than others, but you don't see the one answer choice that is obviously correct. What do you do?

The scenario described above is very common, yet most test takers have not effectively prepared for it. Developing and practicing a plan for guessing may be one of the single most effective uses of your time as you get ready for the exam.

In developing your plan for guessing, there are three questions to address:

- When should you start the guessing process?
- How should you narrow down the choices?
- Which answer should you choose?

When to Start the Guessing Process

Unless your plan for guessing is to select C every time (which, despite its merits, is not what we recommend), you need to leave yourself enough time to apply your answer elimination strategies. Since you have a limited amount of time for each question, that means that if you're going to give yourself the best shot at guessing correctly, you have to decide quickly whether or not you will guess.

Of course, the best-case scenario is that you don't have to guess at all, so first, see if you can answer the question based on your knowledge of the subject and basic reasoning skills. Focus on the key words in the question and try to jog your memory of related topics. Give yourself a chance to bring the knowledge to mind, but once you realize that you don't have (or you can't access) the knowledge you need to answer the question, it's time to start the guessing process.

It's almost always better to start the guessing process too early than too late. It only takes a few seconds to remember something and answer the question from knowledge. Carefully eliminating wrong answer choices takes longer. Plus, going through the process of eliminating answer choices can actually help jog your memory.

Summary: Start the guessing process as soon as you decide that you can't answer the question based on your knowledge.

7

How to Narrow Down the Choices

The next chapter in this book (**Test-Taking Strategies**) includes a wide range of strategies for how to approach questions and how to look for answer choices to eliminate. You will definitely want to read those carefully, practice them, and figure out which ones work best for you. Here though, we're going to address a mindset rather than a particular strategy.

Your chances of guessing an answer correctly depend on how many options you are choosing from.

How many choices you have	How likely you are to guess correctly
5	20%
4	25%
3	33%
2	50%
1	100%

You can see from this chart just how valuable it is to be able to eliminate incorrect answers and make an educated guess, but there are two things that many test takers do that cause them to miss out on the benefits of guessing:

- Accidentally eliminating the correct answer
- Selecting an answer based on an impression

We'll look at the first one here, and the second one in the next section.

To avoid accidentally eliminating the correct answer, we recommend a thought exercise called **the $5 challenge**. In this challenge, you only eliminate an answer choice from contention if you are willing to bet $5 on it being wrong. Why $5? Five dollars is a small but not insignificant amount of money. It's an amount you could afford to lose but wouldn't want to throw away. And while losing $5 once might not hurt too much, doing it twenty times will set you back $100. In the same way, each small decision you make—eliminating a choice here, guessing on a question there—won't by itself impact your score very much, but when you put them all together, they can make a big difference. By holding each answer choice elimination decision to a higher standard, you can reduce the risk of accidentally eliminating the correct answer.

The $5 challenge can also be applied in a positive sense: If you are willing to bet $5 that an answer choice *is* correct, go ahead and mark it as correct.

Summary: Only eliminate an answer choice if you are willing to bet $5 that it is wrong.

Which Answer to Choose

You're taking the test. You've run into a hard question and decided you'll have to guess. You've eliminated all the answer choices you're willing to bet $5 on. Now you have to pick an answer. Why do we even need to talk about this? Why can't you just pick whichever one you feel like when the time comes?

The answer to these questions is that if you don't come into the test with a plan, you'll rely on your impression to select an answer choice, and if you do that, you risk falling into a trap. The test writers know that everyone who takes their test will be guessing on some of the questions, so they intentionally write wrong answer choices to seem plausible. You still have to pick an answer though, and if the wrong answer choices are designed to look right, how can you ever be sure that you're not falling for their trap? The best solution we've found to this dilemma is to take the decision out of your hands entirely. Here is the process we recommend:

Once you've eliminated any choices that you are confident (willing to bet $5) are wrong, select the first remaining choice as your answer.

Whether you choose to select the first remaining choice, the second, or the last, the important thing is that you use some preselected standard. Using this approach guarantees that you will not be enticed into selecting an answer choice that looks right, because you are not basing your decision on how the answer choices look.

This is not meant to make you question your knowledge. Instead, it is to help you recognize the difference between your knowledge and your impressions. There's a huge difference between thinking an answer is right because of what you know, and thinking an answer is right because it looks or sounds like it should be right.

Summary: To ensure that your selection is appropriately random, make a predetermined selection from among all answer choices you have not eliminated.

9

Test-Taking Strategies

This section contains a list of test-taking strategies that you may find helpful as you work through the test. By taking what you know and applying logical thought, you can maximize your chances of answering any question correctly!

It is very important to realize that every question is different and every person is different: no single strategy will work on every question, and no single strategy will work for every person. That's why we've included all of them here, so you can try them out and determine which ones work best for different types of questions and which ones work best for you.

Question Strategies

Read Carefully

Read the question and answer choices carefully. Don't miss the question because you misread the terms. You have plenty of time to read each question thoroughly and make sure you understand what is being asked. Yet a happy medium must be attained, so don't waste too much time. You must read carefully, but efficiently.

Contextual Clues

Look for contextual clues. If the question includes a word you are not familiar with, look at the immediate context for some indication of what the word might mean. Contextual clues can often give you all the information you need to decipher the meaning of an unfamiliar word. Even if you can't determine the meaning, you may be able to narrow down the possibilities enough to make a solid guess at the answer to the question.

Prefixes

If you're having trouble with a word in the question or answer choices, try dissecting it. Take advantage of every clue that the word might include. Prefixes and suffixes can be a huge help. Usually they allow you to determine a basic meaning. Pre- means before, post- means after, pro - is positive, de- is negative. From prefixes and suffixes, you can get an idea of the general meaning of the word and try to put it into context.

Hedge Words

Watch out for critical hedge words, such as *likely, may, can, sometimes, often, almost, mostly, usually, generally, rarely*, and *sometimes*. Question writers insert these hedge phrases to cover every possibility. Often an answer choice will be wrong simply because it leaves no room for exception. Be on guard for answer choices that have definitive words such as *exactly* and *always*.

Switchback Words

Stay alert for *switchbacks*. These are the words and phrases frequently used to alert you to shifts in thought. The most common switchback words are *but, although*, and *however*. Others include *nevertheless, on the other hand, even though, while, in spite of, despite, regardless of*. Switchback words are important to catch because they can change the direction of the question or an answer choice.

Face Value

When in doubt, use common sense. Accept the situation in the problem at face value. Don't read too much into it. These problems will not require you to make wild assumptions. If you have to go beyond creativity and warp time or space in order to have an answer choice fit the question, then you should move on and consider the other answer choices. These are normal problems rooted in reality. The applicable relationship or explanation may not be readily apparent, but it is there for you to figure out. Use your common sense to interpret anything that isn't clear.

Answer Choice Strategies

Answer Selection

The most thorough way to pick an answer choice is to identify and eliminate wrong answers until only one is left, then confirm it is the correct answer. Sometimes an answer choice may immediately seem right, but be careful. The test writers will usually put more than one reasonable answer choice on each question, so take a second to read all of them and make sure that the other choices are not equally obvious. As long as you have time left, it is better to read every answer choice than to pick the first one that looks right without checking the others.

Answer Choice Families

An answer choice family consists of two (in rare cases, three) answer choices that are very similar in construction and cannot all be true at the same time. If you see two answer choices that are direct opposites or parallels, one of them is usually the correct answer. For instance, if one answer choice says that quantity x increases and another either says that quantity x decreases (opposite) or says that quantity y increases (parallel), then those answer choices would fall into the same family. An answer choice that doesn't match the construction of the answer choice family is more likely to be incorrect. Most questions will not have answer choice families, but when they do appear, you should be prepared to recognize them.

Eliminate Answers

Eliminate answer choices as soon as you realize they are wrong, but make sure you consider all possibilities. If you are eliminating answer choices and realize that the last one you are left with is also wrong, don't panic. Start over and consider each choice again. There may be something you missed the first time that you will realize on the second pass.

Avoid Fact Traps

Don't be distracted by an answer choice that is factually true but doesn't answer the question. You are looking for the choice that answers the question. Stay focused on what the question is asking for so you don't accidentally pick an answer that is true but incorrect. Always go back to the question and make sure the answer choice you've selected actually answers the question and is not merely a true statement.

Extreme Statements

In general, you should avoid answers that put forth extreme actions as standard practice or proclaim controversial ideas as established fact. An answer choice that states the "process should be used in certain situations, if..." is much more likely to be correct than one that states the "process should be discontinued completely." The first is a calm rational statement and doesn't even make a

11

definitive, uncompromising stance, using a hedge word *if* to provide wiggle room, whereas the second choice is a radical idea and far more extreme.

Benchmark

As you read through the answer choices and you come across one that seems to answer the question well, mentally select that answer choice. This is not your final answer, but it's the one that will help you evaluate the other answer choices. The one that you selected is your benchmark or standard for judging each of the other answer choices. Every other answer choice must be compared to your benchmark. That choice is correct until proven otherwise by another answer choice beating it. If you find a better answer, then that one becomes your new benchmark. Once you've decided that no other choice answers the question as well as your benchmark, you have your final answer.

Predict the Answer

Before you even start looking at the answer choices, it is often best to try to predict the answer. When you come up with the answer on your own, it is easier to avoid distractions and traps because you will know exactly what to look for. The right answer choice is unlikely to be word-for-word what you came up with, but it should be a close match. Even if you are confident that you have the right answer, you should still take the time to read each option before moving on.

General Strategies

Tough Questions

If you are stumped on a problem or it appears too hard or too difficult, don't waste time. Move on! Remember though, if you can quickly check for obviously incorrect answer choices, your chances of guessing correctly are greatly improved. Before you completely give up, at least try to knock out a couple of possible answers. Eliminate what you can and then guess at the remaining answer choices before moving on.

Check Your Work

Since you will probably not know every term listed and the answer to every question, it is important that you get credit for the ones that you do know. Don't miss any questions through careless mistakes. If at all possible, try to take a second to look back over your answer selection and make sure you've selected the correct answer choice and haven't made a costly careless mistake (such as marking an answer choice that you didn't mean to mark). This quick double check should more than pay for itself in caught mistakes for the time it costs.

Pace Yourself

It's easy to be overwhelmed when you're looking at a page full of questions; your mind is confused and full of random thoughts, and the clock is ticking down faster than you would like. Calm down and maintain the pace that you have set for yourself. Especially as you get down to the last few minutes of the test, don't let the small numbers on the clock make you panic. As long as you are on track by monitoring your pace, you are guaranteed to have time for each question.

Don't Rush

It is very easy to make errors when you are in a hurry. Maintaining a fast pace in answering questions is pointless if it makes you miss questions that you would have gotten right otherwise. Test writers like to include distracting information and wrong answers that seem right. Taking a little extra time to avoid careless mistakes can make all the difference in your test score. Find a pace that allows you to be confident in the answers that you select.

Keep Moving

Panicking will not help you pass the test, so do your best to stay calm and keep moving. Taking deep breaths and going through the answer elimination steps you practiced can help to break through a stress barrier and keep your pace.

Final Notes

The combination of a solid foundation of content knowledge and the confidence that comes from practicing your plan for applying that knowledge is the key to maximizing your performance on test day. As your foundation of content knowledge is built up and strengthened, you'll find that the strategies included in this chapter become more and more effective in helping you quickly sift through the distractions and traps of the test to isolate the correct answer.

Now it's time to move on to the test content chapters of this book, but be sure to keep your goal in mind. As you read, think about how you will be able to apply this information on the test. If you've already seen sample questions for the test and you have an idea of the question format and style, try to come up with questions of your own that you can answer based on what you're reading. This will give you valuable practice applying your knowledge in the same ways you can expect to on test day.

Good luck and good studying!

14

Health Maintenance and Promotion

Growth and Development

Growth and Development During Infancy

<u>First Month</u>

The newborn sleeps about 16 hours/day during the **first month** but is growing and developing:

- *Growth:* Infants lose 5-7% of birth weight and then gain 4-7 ounces per week (about 2 lbs/month). Head circumference increases 1.5cm/month and length 1.5 cm/month.
- *Mobility:* The infant makes fists and flexes arms and legs. Reflexes such as Moro, sucking, grasping, startle, rooting, and asymmetric tonic neck are present.
- *Feeding:* About every 2-3 hours with breastfeeding.
- *Urine/feces:* Urination is about 8 times/day. Breastfed babies may have frequent loose stools or may skip 2-3 days. If bottle-fed, stools are usually more firm. Color varies (yellow, tan, green, brown).
- *Sensory:* Follows items in line of vision and often prefers faces and contrasting geometric designs. Vision is somewhat blurry with ability to focus at about 8-15 inches. Color distinction is poor. Babies hear well and respond with startle reflex. Sense of smell is strong.
- *Communication:* Infant signals distress with crying, gagging, and arching body and respond to comfort measures.

<u>2-4 Months</u>

During **months 2-4,** the infant continues to sleep much of the time but is often awake for periods in the morning, afternoon, and evening:

- *Growth:* Gains 5-7 ounces/week and 1.5 cm length/month and 1.5cm head circumference/month. Posterior fontanel closes.
- *Mobility:* Loses grasp reflex and hands start to stay open and grasp. Able to lift head while prone or supine and turn from side to side. Can roll stomach to back by 4 months. Moro reflex fades. Plays with hands.
- *Feeding:* Needs about 2 oz/lb/24 hours, usually feeding every 4 hours. Can be pulled to standing position.
- *Urine/feces:* Urine is about 5-6 times/day. Stools vary from one each feeding to every 2-3 days, but usually are more firm and regular.
- *Sensory:* Can focus at about 12 inches and follows objects 180° with eyes.
- *Communication:* Crying differentiates to show hunger, pain, frustration. Infant can smile indiscriminately by 2 months and has a socially responsive smile by 3 months. Child shows preference for mother and may turn from strangers.

15

4-6 Months

During **4-6 months** the child sleeps about 10-11 hours at night, with 2-3 daytime naps (total 15 hours).

- *Growth:* Doubles weight by 5-6 months, 5-7 oz/week.
- *Mobility:* Infant can roll over and roll from back to side by 6 months and can hold head up at 90° and turn head in both directions when sitting or lying. Can sit with support for 10-15 minutes. Grasp improves and may hold bottle and play with feet. By 6 months, can pick up items and move items from one hand to the other. Manipulates and mouths objects and watches objects fall.
- *Feeding:* Still having about 2 feedings at night and every 4 hours during the day, 1.5 oz/lb/ per 24 hours.
- *Urine/feces:* Urination and defecation becoming regular.
- *Sensory:* Eyes focus well and follows items/people with eyes.
- *Communication:* Vocalizing more and mimicking tones. Squeals and laughs. Yells with anger. Vocalizes to get attention and recognizes family members.

6-8 Months

During **6-8 months** the child begins to have more waking hours, sleeping 10-11 hours with 2 naps:

- *Growth:* Growth slows. Gains 3-5 oz/wk and 1cm in length/month.
- *Mobility:* Can sit alone by 8 months. Can stand supported and bounces on legs. Starting to use pincer grasp. Easily manipulates and moves objects. Most birth reflexes have faded. Bangs objects together and mouths objects freely.
- *Feeding:* Starting to take solid foods (cereal, vegetables, fruit) 2-3 times daily as well as breastfeeding/bottle-feeding 3-5 times daily. Teething biscuits, graham crackers, and Melba toast may be introduced.
- *Urine/feces:* Stool larger with solid foods. Urinating 5-6 times daily.
- *Sensory:* Watches and listens actively, turning head to sounds and to follow objects.
- *Communication:* Increased babbling and mimicking of sounds, including two syllable sounds and vowels, such as "mama" or "dada" but doesn't use intentionally. Has babbling conversations. May be fearful of strangers.

8-10 Months

During **8-10 months,** the child continues to sleep about 10-11 hours at night and usually sleeps through the night, with 2 naps in the daytime:

- *Growth:* Gains 3-5 oz/wk and 1 cm in length/month.
- *Mobility:* Uses pincer grasp well and can pick up small objects. Crawls or creeps readily. Can sit up and by 10 months can pull to standing position by holding onto furniture.
- *Feeding:* Meat is introduced. Breastfeeding or bottle-feeding 3-4 times daily with 3 meals. Eggs yolks only may be introduced. Will enjoy finger foods, such as meat sticks.
- *Urine/feces:* Fairly regular.
- *Sensory:* Watches and listens freely, attentive.
- *Communication:* Babbles and may be able to say one or two words besides "mama" or "dada." Understands basic vocabulary, such as "no" and "cookie." Babbling follows speech like rhythm when "talking."

10-12 Months

During **10-12 months**, the child continues to sleep 10-11 hours at night with 2 naps in the daytime:

- *Growth:* Gains 3-5 ounces a week and 1 cm/month. Head and chest circumference are equal. Birth weight tripled by 12 months.
- *Mobility:* Can make marks on paper with pens or crayons. Fits objects through holes. Can stand alone and walk holding onto furniture. Can sit from standing position.
- *Feeding:* Breastfeeding or bottle-feeding 3-4 times daily and starting with "sippy" cup. Eating solid foods, both prepared baby foods and soft home-cooked foods. Enjoys finger foods and may resist being fed.
- *Urine/feces:* May smear feces. Holding urine for longer periods of time, especially girls.
- *Sensory:* Watches and listens, engaging in activities.
- *Communication:* Understands many words. Uses "mama" and "dada" intentionally and may use a few other words. Plays patty-cake and peek-a-boo games. Enjoys repetition.

1-2 Years

Between **1 and 2,** the child is growing in size and independence:

- *Growth:* Gains 8 oz/month and 3-5 in/year. Anterior fontanel closes.
- *Mobility:* Begins with first steps and by 2 walks and runs and can go up and down stairs. Scribbles on paper, throws toys, learns to stack blocks. Begins independent exploration of environment.
- *Diet:* Child eats 3 meals and 2-3 snacks daily. Whole cow's milk can be taken after 1 year, 2-3 cups daily. Some may breastfeed. Child can consume wide range of foods.
- *Toileting:* Between 18-24 months, some children show an interest in potty training.
- *Communication:* Begins with one word and grows. Learns names for common objects and begins trying to communicate with simple words leading to short sentences around 2 with vocabulary of 30-50 words. May show apprehension with strangers and anger with temper tantrums.

2-3 Years

The **2-3-year-old** makes significant changes over the course of a year:

- *Growth:* Gains 3-5 lb/year and 3.5-5 in/year.
- *Mobility:* Can run steadily, jump on two feet, and climb. Scribbling becomes more intentional and can draw simple shapes. Makes effort to color in the lines. Able to undress at 2 and dress at 3. Can throw a ball overhand. Plays side by side and begins to interact with others.
- *Diet:* Child can switch to low fat milk, 2-3 cups daily along with a regular well-balanced meal of meat, fruits, vegetables, and grains. Should limit fruit juice to 2-4 oz/day because of high sugar content. Should not be receiving bottle feedings.
- *Toileting:* Most children become potty-trained some time during this year.
- *Communication/cognition:* Child begins to talk in short 3-word sentences and to understand rules. Begins to use pronouns (I, me, you) and can talk about feelings. Usually knows at least 5 body parts and colors and can categorize by size (big, little).

Growth and Development During Preschool Years

From ages **3-6,** the child moves from being a toddler to a child:

- *Growth:* Gains 3-5 lb/yr and 1.5-2.5 in/year. Most growth occurs in long bones as child increases in stature and proportionate head size decreases.
- *Mobility:* Becomes increasingly adept, drawing various shapes, coloring in the lines, using scissors to cut along lines. Can brush teeth. Can tie shoes by 6. Able to climb, run, jump, balance, and ride tricycle or bicycle with training wheels. Interacts with others.
- *Diet:* Eats 3 meals with snack and can manage spoon, fork, and knife independently by age 6.
- *Communication/cognition:* Becomes increasingly verbal and social and commands a large complex vocabulary by 6. Understands concepts of right and wrong, good and bad, and can lie. Learns letters and numbers and by age 6 is beginning to read. May focus on one thing to the exclusion of others.

Growth and Development Problems During School-Age Years

During the years of **6-12,** routine health assessments should be done at ages 6, 8, 10, 11, and 12 to determine if there are developmental delays or problems, which may include:

- *6 years:* Peer problems, depression, cruelty to animals, poor academic progress, speech problems, lack of fine motor skills, and inability to catch a ball or state age.
- *8 years:* No close friends, depression, cruelty to animals, interest in fires, very poor academic progress with inability to do math, read, or write adequately and poor coordination.
- *10 years:* No team sports and poor choices in peers (gangs), failure to follow rules, cruelty to animals and interest in fires, depression, failure to understand causal relationships, poor academic progress in reading, writing, math, and penmanship, and problem throwing or catching.
- *12 years:* Continuation of problems at 10 years with increasing risk-taking behaviors (drinking, drugs, sex) and continued poor academic progress in reading, following directions, doing homework, and organization.

Growth and Development Issues for Early Adolescence

Early adolescence, **11-14,** is a transitional time for children as their hormones and their bodies go through changes. Children mature at varying rates, so there are wide differences. Emotions may be labile, and the child may feel isolated and confused at times, trying to find an identity. Peers take on more influence and the child may challenge the values of the family. Children may have much anxiety about their bodies and sexuality as secondary sexual characteristics develops. Developmental concerns include:

- Delayed maturation.
- Short stature (female).
- Spinal curvature (females).
- Poor dental status (caries, malocclusion).
- Chronic illnesses, such as diabetes.
- Lack of adequate physical activity.
- Poor nutrition, anorexia.
- Concerns about sexual identity.
- Negative self-image.

- Depression.
- Lack of close friends.
- Fighting or violent episodes.
- Poor academic progress with truancy and failure to complete assignments.
- Lack of impulse control.
- Obesity.

Normal Growth and Development Issues for Middle Adolescence

In middle adolescence, ages **15-17,** most body changes have occurred, and there is less concern about this but more concern about the image they are projecting. Girls may worry about weight and boys about muscle development. May be interested in sexuality and many begin sexual experimentation. They identify with peer groups, including codes of dress and behavior, often putting them at odds with family. Developmental concerns are:

- Spinal curvature and short stature (males).
- Lack of testicular maturation/ persistent gynecomastia.
- Acne. Anorexia and Obesity.
- Sexual experimentation, multiple partners, and unprotected sex.
- Sexual identification concerns.
- Depression. Poor self-image.
- Lack of adequate exercise.
- Poor nutrition and poor dental health.
- Chronic diseases.
- Experimentation with drugs and alcohol.
- Problems with authority figures.
- Lack of peer group identification.
- Gang association.
- Poor academic progress, failing classes, truancy, attention deficits and disruptive class behavior.
- Poor judgment and impulse control.

Normal Growth and Development Issues for Late Adolescence

Late adolescence, **18-21,** is the time when adolescents begin to take on more adult roles and responsibilities, entering the world of work or going to college. Most have come to terms with their sexuality and have a more mature understanding of people's motivations. Some young people will continue to engage in high-risk behaviors. Many of the problems associated with middle adolescence may continue if unresolved, interfering with the transition to adulthood. Developmental concerns include:

- Failure to take on adult roles, no life goals or future plans.
- Low self-esteem.
- Lack of intimate relationships.
- Sexual identification concerns.
- Gang association.
- Continued identification with peer group or dependence on parents.
- High-risk sexual behavior, multiple partners and unprotected sex.
- Depression.
- Poor academic progress or ability.

- Psychosomatic complaints.
- Lack of impulse control.
- Poor nutrition. Poor dental health.
- Chronic disease.
- Obesity. Lack of exercise.

Maturity Assessment

A **maturity assessment** should be part of the preparticipation examination for children and adolescents to determine their level of sexual, dental, and skeletal maturity:

- **Skeletal maturity** is usually assessed by measurements of the hand and wrist and well as weight/height for age. Skeletal maturity and chronological age may differ. For example, if the chronological age is 14.3 and the skeletal age is 15.5, this would be expressed as 15.5-14.3=SA+1.2. Another method is to divide the skeletal age by the chronological age: a score >1.0 equates with advanced skeletal maturity and <1 a delay in skeletal maturity.
- The most common assessment tool for **sexual maturity** is Tanner's 5 stages of assessment. This tool assesses maturity for both males and females, based on direct observation of breasts and genitals:
- Females: breast development, onset of menses, and pubic hair distribution.
- Males: Penis and testes development and pubic hair distribution.

Anticipatory Guidance

Children/Families

Providing **anticipatory guidance** to children/families is an important role for the APRN, who is guided by knowledge about risk factors and growth and development. As the child moves from one stage of development to another, the nurse should provide information first to the parents and then to the parents and child about what to expect in terms of development, both physically and emotionally as well as how to minimize risk factors. Guidance may be related to a number of different areas of concern:

- Diet and nutrition, especially for those children at risk for obesity or eating disorders.
- Safety measures, including information about common types of childhood injuries.
- Sexual development and normal related changes and behaviors.
- Sports activities and exercise that is age-appropriate,
- General growth and development.
- Academic progress, and advice about testing and intervention for learning disabilities.
- Peer influence.
- Drug and alcohol abuse.

Early Adolescence

Children during early adolescence (11-14) are undergoing many changes in their bodies and emotions. Relationships with family and peers may begin to change, and the child may be very self-conscious and concerned that they are normal. **Anticipatory guidance** helps the child to navigate changes in his/her life and to negotiate changes in relationships as the child seeks more autonomy:

- *Physical changes:* Outline what the child should expect in terms of bodily changes, such as development of secondary sexual characteristics, including normal variations, and height and weight changes.
- *Cognitive changes:* Allow the child to express changes in thought patterns and awareness and discuss how that relates to developing maturity and stress the importance of maintaining academic responsibilities.
- *Socio-behavioral changes:* Ask the child about peer groups and pressures at school and discuss methods to avoid gangs, tobacco, drugs, and alcohol, and abusive relationship.

Middle Adolescence

Middle adolescence (15-17) is a time of conflict for many young people as they strive to establish an identity separate from their parents and at the same time fit in and find acceptance with their peers. For many, this is the most difficult time of adolescence, and the APRN should provide **anticipatory guidance** to the adolescent through this time, even if the adolescent appears uninterested. Adolescents want respect and often respond when treated with respect. Encouraging the adolescent to discuss issues is more productive that providing direct guidance:

- *Physical changes:* Discuss the responsibilities that come with sexual maturity, including abstinence or birth control. Demonstrate breast and testicular self-examinations.
- *Cognitive changes:* Discuss future goals, both life plans and academic plans, providing guidance in relation to steps the adolescent needs to take in order to meet those goals.
- *Sociobehavioral changes:* Discuss relationships and risk-taking behavior while focusing on means to increase safety.

Nutrition Guidelines

Nutrition in Infants

1-6 Months

Breast milk provides the best **nutrition** for infants and breastfeeding should be encouraged for all mothers during the child's **first year**, with solid food added during the last 6 months. If formula is used, it should be iron-fortified for the first year. Cow's milk must be avoided until after 1 year because it can cause bleeding and anemia because of immaturity of the digestive tract.

- *First month:* Eats about every 2-3 hours, taking 60-90 mL per feeding.
- *2-4 months:* Eats about every 3-4 hours, taking 90-120 mL per feeding.
- *4-6 months:* Eats 4-5 times daily, taking 100-150 mL per feeding. Often begins rice cereal at 4 months, 1-2 tablespoons 1-2 times daily before formula or breastfeeding, increasing to 1/4 cup 2 times daily by 6 months. Rice cereal contains iron and has low allergic potential and is easy to digest.

6-12 Months

As the child begins to eat other foods at **6-12 months**, milk must remain part of the **nutrition**, either breast milk or iron-fortified formula:

- *6-8 months:* Eats 4 times daily, 160-225 mL per feeding. Now having rice cereal, fruits, and vegetables with meals, with foods introduced one at a time about ≥3 days apart to observe for allergies.
- *8-10 months:* Eats 4 times daily, taking 160 mL per feeding. Meats may gradually be added at this time, but are harder to digest and may cause indigestion in some children. Eats finger foods, such as soft pieces of vegetables, cheese, tofu, cereals and meat sticks.
- *10-12 months:* Eats 4 times daily, taking about 160-225 mL per feeding. Usually weaning from breast or bottle and begins using "sippy" cup with lid. Is able to eat most soft foods with rest of the family and continues to enjoy finger foods. Makes attempts to self-feed with spoon.

Nutrition for Toddlers and Preschoolers

Growth begins to slow for the **toddler and preschooler**, but nutritional demands remain high because of the child's increased size and activity. During these years, children still need milk, but intake should not exceed 1 quart daily. Children usually eat 3 meals and 2 snacks, the same foods as the rest of the family, learning eating habits from parents. Two different phenomena may occur:

- *Physiologic anorexia* occurs when high metabolic demands of infancy slow and toddlers may have periods when they eat little, but if intake is averaged over days or weeks, it is adequate.
- *Food jags* are common with preschoolers, days or even weeks when they refuse all but one or two foods. Studies have indicated that children seem to suffer no ill effects, so forcing the child to eat other food isn't necessary, but other foods should be offered until child resumes a more normal diet.

Common Diet Deficiencies in Infants and Children

While poor nutritional intake can result in a number of different **dietary deficiencies**, some are more common in infants and children:

- *Calcium:* Calcium is essential for the growth and development of bones, but children, especially teenagers, are increasingly substituting fruit juice and sodas for milk. This can cause fractures and osteomalacia with eventual osteoporosis as an adult. Recommended daily intake for adolescents is 1500mg.
- *Folic acid:* Intake is often low among teenagers, resulting in high rates of congenital abnormalities if they get pregnant. Cereals and breads are fortified with folic acid to combat this.
- *Iron:* Newborns deplete their maternally-supplied iron by about 4 months and may become anemic if breast-fed without supplementary rice cereal. Formula is iron-fortified. Teenage girls are also often iron-deficient because of menses and poor dietary intake.
- *Vitamin D:* Deficiencies are on the rise because of judicious use of sunscreen and protecting children from all sun exposure. Breast-fed infants may need Vitamin D supplements.

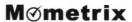

Dietary Management of Obesity in Children

Obesity in children and teenagers is increasing with 16-33% classified as overweight. While there is no clear agreement about weight standards for children, excess weight is having a profound effect on children's health. However, helping the child to lose weight can be difficult:

- Dieting is best approached as a healthier change in eating habits for the whole family so that the child does not eat differently from others.
- No more than 30% of nutrition should be fats.
- Carbohydrates should be complex rather than simple sugars, decreasing consumption of white flour and sugar.
- Healthy snacks, such as fruit, air-popped popcorn, and nonfat yogurt, should be provided with high-caloric snacks (chips, candy) not available.
- The child should eat 3 meals daily, served adequate but not large portions, and not be forced to "clean the plate."
- Television viewing or other sedentary activities should be progressively limited over time and exercise activities encouraged.

Adverse Food Reactions

Adverse food reactions include both allergies and food intolerances:

- *Allergies* cause an immune response, which may be almost instantaneous upon ingestion or contact with a food, or delayed reactions, which may occur hours later:
  - Mild reactions may begin with localized swelling or itching.
  - Stronger reactions may result in generalized erythema and edema, increasing to mild wheezing and laryngeal edema.
  - Severe anaphylactic reactions result in hypotension, severe dyspnea, and cardiac and respiratory arrest.
- The foods implicated in 90% of food allergies are cow's milk, peanuts, tree nuts, eggs, soya, wheat, fish, and shellfish.
- *Intolerance* is the inability of the body to metabolize foods or food products and is a nonimmunologic response. Common intolerances are those related to enzyme deficiencies, such as lactose intolerance, or the inability to metabolize various other biochemicals, such as food additives. Some intolerances are related to gastrointestinal abnormalities, such as cystic fibrosis, and others to psychological problems.

Sun Exposure

For many years, parents were advised to protect children from all **sun exposure** in order to prevent skin damage that could lead to skin cancer, but this, and a decrease in milk drinking, has resulted in increasing evidence of vitamin D deficiency and even an increase in cases of rickets. This is fueling a debate between physicians who believe that some sun exposure is warranted for children and others who insist that all exposure is harmful. Recent guidelines suggest that approximately 20 minutes of sun exposure daily with arms exposed, avoiding direct mid-day sun from 10-2 PM (when UV levels are below 3) and burns, is a safe amount of time and will prevent vitamin D deficiency. Dark-skinned children may tolerate more time in the sun without burning. For longer periods of time, sunscreen should be applied to all exposed areas of skin, especially in children who are fair and prone to burning.

Exercise

Daily **exercise** is an important component of good health practices but should be age-appropriate, and some health conditions may pose restrictions on types of activities. Toddlers and young children usually get exercise by running and playing and do not need organized activities, but older children and teenagers may benefit from activities such as biking or other sports:

- *4-5-year-olds* may participate in dancing, skating and other supervised activities but lack coordination and judgment about safety.
- *6-12-year-olds* are still growing and muscles are short, so they do best with non-competitive sports, such as bicycling and swimming, until about age 10. Team sports should be supervised to ensure children are not straining muscles. Weight lifting may be done at 11 to build strength. Gymnastics may begin but children should be monitored for eating disorders.
- *12-18-year-olds* can participate in any sports activity unless limited by illness or disability. Exercise should be done at least 3 times weekly for 30 minutes.

Heat-Related Illness

Children are particularly vulnerable to **heat-related illness**, especially when heat is combined with humidity, because of a low ratio of surface area to body mass and less capacity for perspiration. Heat-related illnesses occur when heat accumulation in the body outpaces dissipation, resulting in increased temperature and dehydration, which can then lead to thermoregulatory failure and multiple organ dysfunction syndromes. Each year in the United States, about 29 children die from heat stroke after being left in automobiles. At temperatures of 72-96 °F, the temperature in a car rises 3.2° every 5 minutes, with 80% of rise within 30 minutes. Temperatures can reach 117 °F even on cool days. There are 3 types of heat-related illness:

- *Heat stress:* Increased temperature causes dehydration. Child may develop swelling of hands and feet, itching of skin, sunburn, heat syncope (pale moist skin, hypotension), heat cramps, and heat tetany (respiratory alkalosis). *Treatment* includes removing from heat, cooling, hydrating, and replacing sodium is usually sufficient.
- *Heat exhaustion:* Involves water or sodium depletion, with sodium depletion common in children and teenagers who are not acclimated to heat. Heat exhaustion can result in flu-like aching, nausea and vomiting, headaches, dizziness, and hypotension with cold clammy skin and diaphoresis. Temperature may be normal or elevated <106 °F. *Treatment* to cool the body and replace sodium and fluids must be prompt in order to prevent heat stroke. Careful monitoring is important and reactions may be delayed.
- *Heat stroke:* Involves failure of the thermoregulatory system with temperatures that may exceed 106 °F and can result in seizures, neurological damage, multiple organ failures and death. Exertional heat stroke often occurs in young athletes who engage in strenuous activities in high heat. Young children are susceptible to non-exertional heat stroke from exposure to high heat. Treatment includes evaporative cooling, rehydration, and supportive treatment according to organ involvement.

Infant Co-Sleeping and Room Sharing

While **co-sleeping** (bed sharing) has been the norm for thousands of years and remains so in many cultures, it has been proven to increase the risk for SIDS, suffocation, and breathing difficulties. For this reason, the American Academy of Pediatrics (AAP) does not recommend co-sleeping, but does acknowledge that many parents unintentionally fall asleep with their baby in the bed, most often when a sleep-deprived mother breastfeeds her child in bed at night. While breastfeeding in bed poses this risk, the AAP feels that this option is safer than many of the alternatives (getting up to feed the infant in a chair or on the couch), and therefore continues to recommend breastfeeding in bed overnight. Parents should be advised to keep the bed clear of loose bedding or pillows that could pose the risk of suffocation if mother and baby fall asleep. Additionally, if the mother falls asleep with the baby during or after nighttime feeding, the AAP recommends that she return the infant to its crib as soon as she wakes up.

The **ABC's of infant sleeping** are that the infant should sleep **alone**, on their **back,** in a **crib**, but the AAP advises pediatricians to withhold judgment when supporting parents who are struggling to implement this guidance. In addition to these ABC's, the AAP now recommends that newborns through 6 months should sleep on their own bed/crib in the same room as the parents. This arrangement, called **room sharing**, has been found to reduce the risk of SIDS.

Sleep Patterns

While **sleeping patterns** may vary considerably for older children and teenagers, who often get insufficient sleep, the patterns of sleep for infants are fairly predictable:

- Neonates sleep about 16 hours a day, awakening to eat every 2-3 hours around the clock. Usually infants in the first 1-2 months should not sleep more than 4 hours at a time because they may become dehydrated. By 3 months, daytime sleep decreases to 5.5 hours with 9.5 at night.
- By 6 months, most infants can sleep through the night (10-11 hours) and take two naps during the day (3.5-4 hours).
- Children slowly increase nighttime sleep and average 11-11.5 hours until about age 4-5. Naps, decreasing in duration, usually continue until about age 3 when 1-hour naps are common.
- 6-9-year-old children need 10-11 hours of sleep, decreasing to about 9 in the teen years and 8-9 by age 18.

Immunization

Immunization is the best means to protect children from a number of communicable diseases. Educating parents about the need for vaccinations is an important role for the nurse practitioner. While parents must be advised of potential side effects, many of the major concerns of parents in relation to thimerosal (which is about 50% mercury by weight) and autism and other disorders have not been supported by studies. Since 2000, vaccines have been thimerosal-free, except for influenza, although some may still contain trace amounts. Despite that, the benefits outweigh perceived risks. Vaccines promote 2 types of immunity:

- *Active immunity:* Antigens are given to promote production of antibodies.
- *Passive immunity:* Antibodies derived from another person with resistance are given to the child.

Some vaccines provide immunity throughout life, but others require periodic booster injections. If a child has a severe allergic reaction to one injection in a series, the rest of the series is contraindicated.

Types of Vaccines

There are a number of different types of **vaccines**:

- *Conjugated forms:* An organism is altered and then joined (conjugated) with another substance, such as a protein, to potentiate immune response (such as conjugated Hib).
- *Killed virus vaccines:* The virus has been killed but can still cause an immune response (such as inactivated poliovirus).
- *Live virus vaccines:* The virus is live but in a weakened (attenuated) form so that it doesn't cause the disease but confers immunity (such as measles vaccine).
- *Recombinant forms:* The organism is genetically altered and for example, may use proteins rather than the whole cell to stimulate immunity (such as Hepatitis B and acellular pertussis vaccine).
- *Toxoid:* A toxin (antigen) that has been weakened by the use of heat or chemicals so it is too weak to cause disease but stimulates antibodies.

Hepatitis A Vaccine

Hepatitis A is a contagious virus that causes liver disease and can cause serious morbidity and death. It is spread through the feces of a person who is infected and often causes contamination of food and water. The Hep A vaccine is now recommended for all children at one year of age. It is not licensed for use in younger infants. Two doses are needed:

- 12 months (12-23 months)
- 18 months (or 6 months after previous dose)

Older children and teenagers may receive the two-injection series if they are considered at risk, depending upon lifestyle, such as young males have sex with other males or those using illegal drugs. It is also recommended if outbreaks occur. Adverse reactions are mild and include soreness, headache, anorexia, and malaise although severe allergic reactions can occur as with all vaccines.

Hepatitis B Vaccine

Hepatitis B is transmitted through blood and body fluids, including during birth; therefore, it is now recommended for all newborns as well as all those<18 and those in high risk groups >18. Hepatitis B can cause serious liver disease leading to liver cancer. Three injections of monovalent HepB are required to confer immunity:

- Birth (within 12 hours)
- Between 1-2 months
- ≥24 weeks
- Note: if combination vaccines are given after the birth dose then a dose at 4 months can be given.

If the mother is Hepatitis B positive, the child should be given both the monovalent HepB vaccination as well as HepB immune globulin within 12 hours of birth. Adolescents (11-15) who have not been vaccinated require 2 doses, 4-6 months apart. Adverse reactions include local irritation and fever. Severe allergic reactions can occur to those allergic to baker's yeast.

Rotavirus Vaccine

Rotavirus is a cause of significant morbidity and mortality in children, especially in developing countries. Most children, without vaccination, will suffer from severe diarrhea caused by rotavirus within the first 5 years of life. The new rotavirus vaccine is advised for all infants but should not be initiated after 12 weeks or administered after 32 weeks, so there is a narrow window of opportunity. Three doses are required:

- 2 months (between 6-12 weeks)
- 4 months
- 6 months

An earlier vaccine was withdrawn from the market because it was associated with an increase in intussusception, a disorder in which part of the intestine telescopes inside another. Rates of intussusception in those receiving the current (RotaTeq®) vaccine have been investigated and incidence of intussusception was within the range of normal occurrences with no evidence linking the occurrences to the vaccine.

DTaP Vaccine

Diphtheria and pertussis (whooping cough) are highly contagious bacterial diseases of the upper respiratory tract. Cases of diphtheria are now rare in the United States although it still occurs in some developing countries. There have, however, been recent outbreaks of pertussis in the United States. Tetanus is a bacterial infection contracted through cuts, wounds, and scratches. The **diphtheria, tetanus, and pertussis (DTaP) vaccine** is recommended for all children. DTaP is a newer and safer version of the older DTP vaccine, which is no longer used in the United States. DTaP requires 5 doses:

- 2 months
- 4 months
- 6 months
- 5-18 months
- 4-6 years (or at 11-12 years if booster missed between 4-6)

This vaccine is not licensed for use for children over 7 years old, but a different vaccine (Tdap) is given to those 11-64 in one dose. Adverse reactions can occur, but they are usually mild soreness, fever, and/or nausea. About 1 in 100 children will have high fever (>105 °F) and may develop seizures. Severe allergic responses can occur.

Inactivated Poliovirus Vaccine

Poliomyelitis is a serious viral infection that can cause paralysis and death. Prior to introduction of a vaccine in 1955, there were >20,000 cases of polio in the United States each year. There have been no cases of polio caused by the poliovirus for >20 years in the United States, but it still occurs in some third world countries, so continuing vaccinations is very important. Oral polio vaccine (OPV) is no longer recommended in the United States because it carries a very slight risk of causing the disease (1:2.4 million). Children require 4 doses of injectable polio vaccine (IPV):

- 2 months
- 4 months
- 6-18 months
- 4-6 years (booster dose)

IPV is contraindicated for those who have had a severe reaction to neomycin, streptomycin, or polymyxin B. Rare allergic reactions can occur, but there are almost no serious problems caused by this vaccine.

Varicella Vaccine

Varicella (chickenpox) is a common infectious childhood disease caused by the varicella zoster virus, resulting in fever, rash, and itching, but it can cause skin infections, pneumonia, and neurological damage. After infection, the virus retreats to the nerves by the spinal cord and can reactivate years later, causing herpes zoster (shingles), a significant cause of morbidity in adults. Infection with varicella conveys immunity, but because of associated problems, it is recommended that all children receive varicella vaccine. Two doses are needed:

- 12-15 months
- 4-6 years (or at least 3 months after 1st dose

Children ≥13 years and adults who have never had chickenpox or previously received the vaccine should receive 2 doses at least 28 days apart. Children should not receive the vaccine if they have had a serious allergic reaction to gelatin or neomycin. Most reactions are mild and include soreness, fever, and rash. About 1:1000 may experience febrile seizures. Pneumonia is a very rare reaction.

MMR Vaccine

Measles is a viral disease characterized by fever and rash but can cause pneumonia, seizures, severe neurological damage, and death. Mump is a viral disease that causes fever and swollen glands but can cause deafness, meningitis, and swelling of the testicles. Rubella, also known as German measles) is also a viral disease that can cause rash, fever, and arthritis, but the big danger is that it can cause a woman who is pregnant to miscarry or deliver a child with serious birth defects. The **measles, mumps, and rubella (MMR) vaccine** is given in 2 doses:

- 12-15 months
- 4-6 years

Children can get the injections at any age if they have missed them, but there must be at least 28 days between injections. Children with severe allergic reactions to gelatin or neomycin should not get the injection. Severe adverse reactions are rare, but fever and mild rash are common. Teenagers may have pain and stiffness in joints. Occasional (1:3000) seizures and thrombocytopenia (1:30,000) occur.

HPV Vaccine

Human papillomavirus (HPV) comprises >100 viruses. About 40 are sexually transmitted and invade mucosal tissue, causing genital warts, which are low risk for cancer, or changes in the mucosa, which can lead to cervical cancer. Most HPVs cause little or no symptoms, but they are very

28

common, especially in those 15-25. Over 99% of cervical cancers are caused by HPV and 70% are related to HPVs 16 and 18. The HPV vaccine, Gardasil®, protects against HPVs 6, 11, which cause genital warts, 16, and 18, causing cancer. Protection is only conveyed if the female has not yet been infected with these strains. The vaccine is currently recommended for females under 18 but studies are determining if males and women over 18 can benefit. A series of 3 injections are required over a 6-month period:

- Initial dose 11-12 years (but may be given as young as 9 or ≥18).
- 2 months after 1st dose.
- 6 months after 1st dose.

PCV-7

Heptavalent pneumococcal conjugate vaccine (PCV-7) (Prevnar®) was released for use in the United States in 2001 for treatment of children under 2 years old. It provides immunity to 7 serotypes of *Streptococcus pneumoniae* to protect against invasive pneumococcal disease, such as pneumonia, otitis media, bacteremia, and meningitis. Because children are most at risk ≤1, vaccinations begin early:

Administration is in 4 doses:
- 1st dose: 6-8 weeks.
- 2nd dose: 4 months.
- 3rd dose: 6 months.
- 4th dose: 12-18 months.

Although less effective for older children, PCV-7 has been approved for children between 2 and 5 years of age who are at high risk because of the following conditions:

- Chronic diseases: sickle cell disease, heart disease, lung disease, liver disease.
- Damaged or missing spleen.
- Immunosuppressive disorders: diabetes, cancer.
- Drug therapy: chemotherapy, steroids.

PCV-7 may also be considered for all children ≤ 5, especially those ≤3 and in group day care and in some ethnic groups (Native American, Alaska Natives, and African Americans).

Meningococcal Vaccine

Meningitis is severe bacterial meningitis that can result in severe neurological compromise or death. A number of different serotypes of *meningococci* can cause meningitis and current vaccines protect against 4 types although not against subtype B, which causes about 65% of meningitis cases in children. However, the vaccines provide 85-100% protection against sub-types A, C, Y, and W-135. There are 2 types of vaccine:

- *Meningococcal polysaccharide vaccine (MPSV4)* is made from the outer capsule of the bacteria and is used for children 2-10.
  - One dose is given at 2 years although those at high risk may receive 2 doses, 3 months apart.
  - Under special circumstances, children 3-24 months may receive 2 doses, 3 months apart.

- Meningococcal conjugate vaccine (MCV4) is used for children ≥11 (who have not received MPSV4). One dose is required:
  o 11-12, all children should receive the vaccine.
  o If not previously vaccinated, high school and college freshmen should be vaccinated.
- Side effects are usually only local tenderness.

HIB Vaccine

Haemophilus influenzae **type b (HIB) vaccine** (HibTITER® and PedavaxHIB®) protects against infection with *Haemophilus influenzae,* which can cause serious respiratory infections, pneumonia, meningitis, bacteremia, and pericarditis in children ≤5 years old. *Administration* is as follows:

- 1st dose: 2 months
- 2nd dose: 4 months
- 3rd dose: 6 months (may be required, depending upon the brand of vaccine)
- Last dose: 12-15 months (this booster dose must be given at least 2 months after the earlier doses for those who start at a later age than 2 months.

Children over age 6 usually do not require HIB, but it is recommended for older children and adults some conditions that place them at risk:

- Sickle cell disease.
- HIV/AIDS.
- Bone marrow transplant.
- Chemotherapy for cancer.
- Damaged or missing spleen.

Some chemotherapy drugs, corticosteroids, and other immunosuppressive drugs may interact with the vaccine.

PPV

Pneumococcal polysaccharide-23 vaccine (PPV)(Pneumovax® and Pnu-Immune®) is a vaccine that has been available since 1977 to protect against 23 types of pneumococcal bacteria. It is given to adults ≥65 and children ≥2 years in high-risk groups that include:

- Children with chronic heart, lung, sickle cell disease, diabetes, cirrhosis, alcoholism, and leaks of cerebrospinal fluid.
- Children with lowered immunity from Hodgkin's disease, lymphoma, leukemia, kidney failure, multiple myeloma, nephrotic syndrome, HIV/AIDS, damaged or missing spleen, and organ transplant.

Children ≤2 may not respond to this vaccine and should take PCV-7. *Administration* is as follows:

- One dose is usually all that is required although a second dose may be advised for children with some conditions, such as cancer or organ/bone marrow transplantations.
- If needed a second dose is given 3 years after the first for children ≤10 and 5 years after the first for those ≥10.

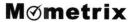

Illness Prevention

Risk Analysis as Part of Disease Prevention

Risk analysis is an important part of health promotion and disease prevention because it can help to identify those factors (normed for age and sex) that put a child at risk for current or future disease. Typically, risk analysis uses observations, interviews and questionnaires to gain information about a child and the family so that interventions and diagnostic testing can be targeted to areas of increased risk. Risk factors may be controllable (diet and exercise) or non-controllable (genetic), but once identified, a plan of care can be formulated. Risk analysis is an important component of cost-containment because early identification and treatment or intervention can reduce future costs of care. Areas for risk analysis may include:

- Nutrition
- Exercise
- Cardiovascular
- Diabetes
- Hypertension
- Cancer
- Osteoporosis
- Vision
- Behavior/lifestyle

Results of risk analysis are not diagnostic, but they indicate if the child is at low, medium, or high risk of developing a disease or health problem.

Elements of Risk Analysis

Risk analysis can be used to assess individual risks or in a broader sense to assess the risk/effectiveness of different treatments and/or programs. Risk analysis should be carried out for all new treatments and procedures to determine if the benefits outweigh the risks and if they are cost-effective Risk analysis should be an ongoing part of the nurse practitioner's role. There are 3 primary components to risk analysis:

- *Assessing* requires gaining information by questioning, observing, or analyzing data, which may be derived from active study or review of the research.
- *Intervening* involves taking information from the assessment and making changes in management, treatments, or procedures to reflect the risk analysis with the aim of providing the most beneficial and cost-effective care.
- *Communicating* requires publishing of results or sharing those with the organization, family, child, or the general public, depending on the scope of the risk analysis.

Risk Factors for Neonates Associated with Maternal Disease/Behavior

There are a number of **maternal factors** that put the infant at increased risk:

- *Diabetes mellitus:* Both gestational and pre-existing diabetes put the infant at risk of stillbirth, hypoglycemia, and macrosomia (larger size than normal) as well as birth injury. Maternal pre-existing diabetes is also associated with birth defects, including abnormal development of the cardiovascular and gastrointestinal systems, neurological and spinal cord disorders, and urinary tract abnormalities.

31

- *Alcohol ingestion:* No safe amount of alcohol for pregnant women has been determined. Infants are at risk for fetal alcohol syndrome that may include facial abnormalities, intellectual disability, and behavioral problems.
- *Tobacco:* Tobacco use causes increased miscarriage, prematurity, and underweight infants.
- *Drug use:* Infants may be born addicted to drugs and go through withdrawal. They may suffer seizure disorders or neurological impairment with long-term learning disabilities.
- *HIV/ Hepatitis B:* Infectious diseases may be transmitted during pregnancy or delivery.

Implications of Fetal Drug Exposure

There are many **drugs** that can profoundly affect the growing fetus. Some are prescribed drugs, such as Accutane®, but the greatest numbers are illicit drugs, such as crack, heroin, or cocaine. Increasing numbers of children are born to addicted mothers. While each drug has specific effects, there are many that are common:

- Premature weight and low birth weight with infants who are small for gestational age (SGA).
- Failure to thrive often related to poor sucking and dysphagia.
- Increased risk of congenital infectious disease (HIV, hepatitis, CMV).
- Increased risk of SIDS.
- Withdrawal symptoms may manifest ≤72 hours after birth:
  o Tremors, excitability, seizures.
  o Vomiting, diarrhea, diaphoresis.
  o Dry, red, irritated skin.
- Developmental and cognitive problems that vary with age. Initial problems often subside within the first couple of years, but in a small number of children learning disabilities and behavioral problems persist.

Implications of Fetal Alcohol Syndrome

Fetal alcohol syndrome (FAS) is a syndrome of birth defects that develop as the result of maternal ingestion of alcohol. Despite campaigns to inform the public, women continue to drink during pregnancy, but no safe amount of alcohol ingestion has been determined. FAS includes:

- *Facial abnormalities:* hypoplastic (underdeveloped) maxilla, micrognathia (undersized jaw), hypoplastic philtrum (groove beneath the nose), short palpebral fissures (eye slits between upper and lower lids).
- *Neurological deficits:* May include microcephaly, intellectual disability, and motor delay, hearing deficits. Learning disorders may include problems with visual-spatial and verbal learning, attention disorders, and delayed reaction times.
- *Growth retardation:* Prenatal growth deficit persists with slow growth after birth.
- *Behavioral problems:* Irritability and hyperactivity. Poor judgment in behavior may relate to deficit in executive functions.

Indication of brain damage without the associated physical abnormalities is referred to as alcohol-related neurodevelopmental disorder (ARND).

Infant Withdrawal from Fetal Exposure to Drugs

Fetal exposure to drugs, such as opioids, methadone, cocaine, crack, and other recreational drugs causes **withdrawal symptoms** in about 60% of infants. There are many variables, which include

32

the type of drug, the extent of drug use, and the duration of maternal drug use. For example, children may have withdrawal symptoms within 48 hours for cocaine, heroin, and methamphetamine exposure, but there may be delays of up to 2 -3weeks for methadone. Short hospital stays after birth make it imperative that children at risk are identified so they can receive supportive treatment, particularly since they often feed poorly and can quickly become dehydrated and undernourished. Polydrug use makes it difficult to describe a typical profile of **symptoms**, but they usually include:

- Tremors.
- Irritability.
- Hypertonicity.
- High-pitched crying.
- Diarrhea.
- Dry skin.
- Seizures (in severe cases).

Treatment is supportive, but children with opiate exposure may be given decreasing doses of opiates, such as morphine elixir, with close monitoring until the child is weaned off of the medication.

Fetal Nicotine/Carbon Monoxide Exposure

About 25% of pregnant women in the United States continue to smoke throughout pregnancy and others are exposed to second-hand smoke, putting the fetus at risk for a number of abnormalities from **exposure to nicotine and carbon monoxide:**

- Fetal growth retardation with damage to neurotransmitters with decrease in number of cells with concomitant damage to peripheral autonomic nervous system.
- Vasoconstriction from nicotine and interference with oxygen transport caused by carbon monoxide can lead to fetal hypoxia.
- Vasoconstriction leading to increased risk of spontaneous abortion, prematurity and low birth weight.
- Increased risk for perinatal death and SIDS.
- Cognitive deficiency and learning disorders, such as auditory processing defects. Children of mothers who smoke have a 50% increase in idiopathic intellectual disability.
- Increased cancer risk, especially for acute lymphocytic leukemia and lymphoma.

Risk Factors for Infants or Children Related to Poverty

Poverty places children at increased risk of stress disorders and disease, especially if children are homeless. The following problems are common:

- *Incomplete or no immunizations* because of lack of health care and regular well-baby or child visits.
- *Frequent infections*, such as respiratory infections or skin infections, because of lack of adequate shelter, living in close quarters, with others, and lack of adequate hygiene.
- *Insufficient sleep*, especially if children are sleeping in cars, on the ground, or in shelters.
- Nutritional deficiencies because of poor diet.
- Dental caries because of poor nutrition and lack of dental care or lack of toothbrushing supplies.
- *Depression* common in all ages.

- Sexual abuse, pregnancies, and sexually transmitted diseases are frequent, especially with homeless teenagers.
- *Injuries* from lack of safety equipment or dangers of the street.

Risk Factors Related to Mental Health Problems in Children and Adolescents

Autism Spectrum Disorders

Autism spectrum disorders (ASD), or pervasive developmental disorders (PDD), affects 3.4:1000 children in the United States and present with a wide range of symptoms, including impairment in thinking and expressions of emotion, using language, and communicating and relating with others. Some children are profoundly impaired and are diagnosed early but more high functioning children, such as those with Asperger's, may go undiagnosed. All exhibit some degree of impairment in 3 areas:

- Social interaction
- Communication (verbal and non-verbal)
- Repetitive behavior

Because they lack social skills, children with ASD are often isolated and bullied. They may do well in school or have some degree of intellectual disability. About 25% suffer from seizure disorders as well. ASD may be identified through developmental screening, and/or specific screening instruments for autism. *Intervention* includes referrals to special education programs, including early intervention programs for children <3 and may include behavioral and speech therapy. Early diagnosis helps maximize the child's potential and may allow the child to live independently as an adult.

ADHD

Mental health problems can interfere with normal growth and development in children and adolescents. Studies indicate that about 10% of children suffer mental disorders that cause some degree of impairment. There are a number of different disorders that affect children. **Attention deficit hyperactivity disorder (ADHD)** affects 2-3% of children. ADHD usually has 3 characteristics:

- Inattention
- Impulsivity
- Hyperactivity

These make it difficult for the child to pay attention in school and keep track of assignments and often results in behavioral and social problems. Additionally, ADHD may be accompanied by learning disabilities, such as dyslexia, as well as depression or other mood disorders. Diagnosis often includes observation and surveys of family and teachers to determine patterns of behavior. *Intervention* includes medications and coping and organizing skills. Studies of different treatments indicate that a combined approach with medications and behavioral therapy is more effective than either medication alone or behavioral therapy alone. The combined approach may allow lower medication dosages.

Borderline Personality Disorder

Borderline personality disorder (BPD) affects about 2% of adults, mostly young women, but symptoms may begin to develop slowly from about 9 and on into the teen years resulting in unstable moods and disordered thinking in relation to self-image and behavior. Self-injury, including self-mutilation, and suicide attempts are common as are drinking and drug use. They may perceive themselves as bad and suffer severe separation anxiety and fears. They often engage in impulsive high-risk behaviors, such as promiscuous sex, and binge eating. Studies have linked BPD to child and sexual abuse as children, with 40-71% of young women diagnosed with BPD victims of sexual abuse during childhood. While definitive diagnosis is usually delayed until young adulthood, because of the associated social and behavioral problems, early recognition of the symptoms and *intervention* with medications and/or behavioral therapy may help the person to cope and develop better behavioral strategies.

Bipolar Disorder

Bipolar disorder causes severe mood swings between hyperactive states and depression, accompanied by impaired judgment because of distorted thoughts. The hypomanic stage may allow for creativity and good functioning in some young people, but it can develop into more severe mania, which may be associated with psychosis and hallucinations, and then into periods of profound depression. While most cases are diagnosed in late adolescence, there is increasing evidence that some children present with symptoms earlier. Especially at risk are children with a bipolar parent. Bipolar disorder is associated with high rates of suicide, so early diagnosis and treatment is critical. Symptoms may be relatively mild or involve severe rapid-cycling between mania and depression. *Intervention* includes both medications (usually given continually) to prevent cycling and control depression and psychosocial therapy, such as cognitive therapy, which helps children control disordered thought patterns and behavior.

Eating Disorders

Eating disorders are a profound health risk, especially for young girls (although boys may also have eating disorders, often presenting as excessive exercise). Different types include:

- *Anorexia nervosa* affects 0.5-3.7% of females, characterized by profound fear of weight gain and severe restriction of food intake, often accompanied by abuse of diuretics and laxatives, which can cause electrolyte imbalances as well as kidney and bowel disorders and delay or cause cessation of menses. Anorexics may become emaciated and risk death.
- *Bulimia nervosa* affects 1.1-4.2% of females and includes binge eating followed by vomiting often along with diuretics, enemas, and laxatives. Gastric acids can damage the throat and teeth. While bulimics may maintain a normal weight, they are at risk for severe electrolyte imbalances that can be life threatening.
- *Binge eating* affects 2-5% of females and includes grossly overeating, often resulting in obesity, depression, and shame.

Early *intervention* can prevent physical damage but hospitalization and intense therapy may be required for long periods of time to change altered thinking.

Depression

Depression is increasingly recognized as a risk factor for children, manifesting in young children as pretending to have an illness or refusal to go to school and in older children as behavioral problems, negativity, and difficulties at school rather than the more common withdrawal and overt depression of some adults. However, children may feel persistent anxiety and sadness and often have profound fears that something will happen to a parent. Usually changes in behavior become apparent. One study showed that 29% of children with depression had suicidal thoughts, making early diagnosis and *intervention* very important. While there is some concern about antidepressants and children, suicide is a leading cause of death in teenagers, so medications with careful monitoring along with psychotherapy, such as cognitive behavioral therapy, seem to provide the best form of treatment, providing >70% with clinical improvement.

Risk Reduction for Diabetes

There has been a marked increase in **diabetes mellitus** in children, correlating with increasing obesity and lack of exercise. This is especially true for minority children. Until recent years, Type I (insulin-dependent) diabetes was most common in children and Type II was rare, but now 8-45% of children presenting with diabetes have Type II (insulin deficiency), although it may be difficult to determine the type with initial diagnosis. Most cases are diagnosed during puberty when hormone changes affect insulin, but children as young as 4 have been identified. Since obesity is a significant risk, health risk reduction efforts are aimed at improving diet and increasing exercise, but intervention aimed at the whole family is often more effective than tailoring diet and exercise just to the needs of the child. The family should work with a nutritionist. Screening with fasting blood sugar is normally done about every 2 years for those at risk or presenting with symptoms.

Cardiovascular Risk Reduction

Some children are at increased risk of developing **cardiovascular disease**, such as coronary artery disease, including those with diabetes mellitus, Kawasaki disease, and familial hypercholesterolemia, which can cause severe coronary artery disease in ≤10 years. Screening children at risk should begin age 2 and include cholesterol levels to assess for an elevation of low-density lipoprotein (LDL):

- Total cholesterol <170 and LDL <110: Normal diet for age.
- Total cholesterol 170-199 and LDL 110-120: Borderline elevation.
- Total cholesterol >200 with LDL >130: Elevated.

Early dietary intervention to reduce cholesterol and prevent increase in LDLs can significantly reduce morbidity and mortality. Dietary recommendations to reduce LDLs include guidelines provided in the *Therapeutic Lifestyle Changes* diet by the American Heart Association (AHA)(http://www.americanheart.org) for those at risk or with elevated cholesterol.

- ≤30% of diet from fat and <7% from saturated fat, >10% polyunsaturated fat, up to 15% monounsaturated fat,
- ≥55% carbohydrates,
- 15% protein
- <200 mg dietary cholesterol per day.

Wellness Evaluation

A **wellness evaluation** is a complete assessment and report of the general health profile of the child, compiling all available pertinent information. A health profile should include the following:

- Basic measurements, such as height, weight, and head circumference and the percentile ranking for age.
- Vital signs, including pulse, respiration and blood pressure. Body temperature should be included as well.
- Nutrition profile that outlines the child's normal diet and any dietary modifications or adverse reactions, such as allergies or intolerances.

- Mobility/activity level that explains the infant's mobility in accordance to expected development for age. For older children, the type of activities and physical exercise that child engages in and the frequency should be noted.
- Results of any screening tests and, if elective rather than standard, the reason for the test.
- Health promotion/disease prevention activities, including duration, results, and compliance with prescribed interventions.

Early Warning Signs of Emergencies

Apnea of Prematurity

Premature infants (especially those <34 weeks) often exhibit **apnea of prematurity (AOP).** AOP begins at birth and is believed caused by immaturity of the nervous system, improving as the brain matures. It may persist for a 4-8 weeks. There are 3 types of apnea:

- *Central*: no airflow or effort to breathe.
- *Obstructive*: no airflow, but effort to breathe.
- *Mixed*: both central and obstructive elements (75% of AOP).

AOP **symptoms** include:

- Swallowing during apneic periods.
- Apnea >20 seconds or apnea < 20 seconds with bradycardia of 30 beats <normal.
- Oxygen saturation <85% persisting ≥5 seconds.
- Cyanosis.

Treatment includes:

- Tactile stimulation (rubbing limbs or thorax or gently slapping bottoms of feet) or gently lifting the jaw to relieve obstruction.
- Oxygen or bag/mask ventilation for bradycardia and ↓oxygen saturation.
- Continuous positive airway pressure (CPAP) for mixed or obstructive apnea.
- Aminophylline (for central apnea) may increase contractions of diaphragm.

Pneumothorax

Pneumothorax is a leak between the lung tissue and the chest wall so extraneous air is in the pleural space. Types include:

- *Spontaneous/Simple pneumothorax* is a breach of the parietal or visceral pleura, such as when an air-filled bleb on the lung surface ruptures or with a bronchopleural fistula without connection to outside air.
- *Traumatic pneumothorax* is a lacerating wound of the chest wall, such as a gunshot or knife wound. It can also result from invasive procedures, such as thoracentesis or lung biopsies or from barotrauma related to ventilation or chest surgery. Open pneumothorax occurs when air passes in and out, causing the lung to collapse, a sucking sound, and paradoxical movement of the chest wall with respirations.
- *Tension pneumothorax* is similar to traumatic open pneumothorax; however, the air can enter the pleural sac but can't be expelled, causing a pronounced mediastinal shift to the unaffected side with severe compromise of cardiac and respiratory function.

Pulmonary and Thoracic Trauma

The diagnostic procedures and tools used during assessment of **pulmonary and thoracic trauma** will vary according to the type and degree of injury, but may include:

- Thorough physical examination including cardiac and pulmonary status, assessing for any abnormalities.
- Electrocardiogram to assess for cardiac arrhythmias.
- Chest x-ray should be done for all those with injuries to check for fractures, pneumothorax, major injuries, and placement of intubation tubes. X-rays can be taken quickly and with portable equipment so they can be completed quickly during the initial assessment.
- Computerized tomography may be indicated after initial assessment, especially if there is a possibility of damage to the parenchyma of the lungs.
- Oximetry and atrial blood gases as indicated.
- 12-lead electrocardiogram may be needed if there are arrhythmias for more careful observation.
- Echocardiogram should be done if there is apparent cardiac damage.

Aspiration Pneumonia

Aspiration pneumonia may occur as the result of any type of aspiration, including foreign objects. The aspirated material creates an inflammatory response, with the irritated mucous membrane at high risk for bacterial infection secondary to the aspiration. With infants and small children, who are weak or suffer from paralysis, congenital anomalies, or lack adequate cough reflex, the most common causes of aspiration pneumonia are fluid or foods. Children with respiratory stress or crying during feeding can easily aspirate. Talcum powder used during diaper changes is also implicated. Toddlers and young children may aspirate lighter fluids or other hydrocarbon liquids. **Symptoms** are similar to other pneumonia, depending upon the site of inflammation: cough, dyspnea, respiratory distress, cyanosis. **Treatment** includes:

- Antibiotic therapy as indicated.
- Symptomatic respiratory support.
- Preventive methods to avoid aspiration, such as careful feeding and positioning child on the right side after feeding.

Foreign Body Aspiration

Infants and children, especially those weak or ill, are prone to **aspiration of foreign substances** (food, powder, secretions) or objects (dry nuts, candy, popcorn, toys). Small children, especially, tend to put almost anything into their mouths. Round foods, such as candies, hot dogs, or foods not easily chewed, such as apples, carrots, or hard cookies are especially dangerous. **Symptoms** include:

- *Initial*: Severe coughing, gagging, sternal retraction, wheezing. Objects in the larynx may cause inability to breathe or speak and may lead to respiratory arrest. If the aspirant lodges in the bronchus, cough, dyspnea, and wheezing occur.
- *Delayed*: Hours, days, or weeks later, an undetected aspirant may cause an infection distal to the aspirated material. Symptoms depend on the area and extent of the infection.

Aspirated foreign bodies are rarely coughed up and must be removed. **Treatment** includes:

- Laryngoscopy or bronchoscopy for removal of object.
- Antibiotic therapy for secondary infection.
- Symptomatic treatment for respiratory distress as indicated.

Status Asthmaticus

Status asthmaticus is a severe acute attack of asthma that does not respond to conventional therapy, such as inhaled bronchodilators, and progresses to respiratory failure. Asthma occurs in about 10% of children in America and both morbidity and mortality rates, especially in African American children, have increased in recent years with twice as many young children requiring hospitalization. An acute attack of asthma is precipitated by some stimulus, such as an antigen that triggers an allergic response, resulting in an inflammatory cascade that causes edema of the mucous membranes (swollen airway), contraction of smooth muscles (bronchospasm), increased mucus production (cough and obstruction), and hyperinflation of airways (decreased ventilation and shunting). Mast cells and T lymphocytes produce cytokines, which continue the inflammatory response through increased blood flow coupled with vasoconstriction and bronchoconstriction, resulting in fluid leakage from the vasculature. Epithelial cells and cilia are destroyed, exposing nerves and causing hypersensitivity. Sympathetic nervous system receptors in the bronchi stimulate bronchodilation.

Symptoms

The 3 primary **symptoms of asthma** are cough, wheezing, and dyspnea. In cough-variant asthma, a severe cough may be the only symptom, at least initially. The child with status asthmaticus will often present in acute distress, non-responsive to inhaled bronchodilators:

- Airway obstruction.
- Sternal and intercostal retractions.
- Tachypnea and dyspnea.
- Increasing cyanosis.
- Forced prolonged expirations.
- Cardiac decompensation with $\uparrow$ left ventricular afterload and increased pulmonary edema resulting from alveolar-capillary permeability. Hypoxia may trigger an $\uparrow$ in pulmonary vascular resistance with $\uparrow$ right ventricular afterload.
- Pulsus paradoxus (decreased pulse on inspiration and increased on expiration) with extra beats on inspiration detected through auscultation but not detected radially. Blood pressure normally decreases slightly during inspiration, but this response is exaggerated. Pulsus paradoxus indicates increasing severity of asthma.
- Hypoxemia (with impending respiratory failure).
- Hypocapnia followed by hypercapnia (with impending respiratory failure).
- Metabolic acidosis.

Risk Factors Associated with Death

There are a number of **risk factors associated with death** from status asthmaticus. Many of the risk factors relate to poor management of asthma on an ongoing basis so that severe asthma attacks occur repeatedly:

- History of sudden, acute exacerbations of disease.
- Endotracheal intubation/ventilation for previous acute episodes of asthma.

- Prior hospitalization and treatment in intensive care for exacerbation.
- ≥2 hospitalizations for asthma in prior 12 months.
- ≥3 visits to the emergency department for asthma treatment in the prior 12 months.
- Overuse of inhaled β-adrenergic agonists (>2 canisters per month).
- Recent tapering and withdrawal of systemic corticosteroids.
- Cardiovascular co-morbidity.
- Low economic status.
- Residence in urban area.

Economic status and place of residence probably reflect inadequate financial resources to bear the cost medical care and treatments, such as preventive medications.

Indications for Mechanical Ventilation

Mechanical ventilation should be avoided if possible because of the danger of increased bronchospasm as well as barotrauma and decreased circulation. Aggressive medical management with β-adrenergic agonists, corticosteroids, and anticholinergics should be tried prior to ventilation. However, there are some absolute indications for the use of intubation and ventilation:

- Cardiac and/or pulmonary arrest.
- Markedly depressed mental status (obtundation).
- Severe hypoxia and/or apnea.
- Bradycardia.

There are a number of other indications that are evaluated on an individual basis and may be an indication for ventilation:

- Exhaustion/ muscle fatigue from exertion of trying to breathe.
- Sharply diminished breath sounds and no audible wheezing.
- Pulse paradoxus >20-40 mm Hg. If pulse paradoxus is absent, this is an indication of imminent respiratory arrest.
- PaO_2 <70 mm Hg on 100% oxygen.
- Deteriorating mental status.
- Dysphonia.
- Central cyanosis.
- ↑Hypercapnia.
- Metabolic/respiratory acidosis; pH <7.20.

Croup Syndromes

Croup is not a disease in itself but rather a syndrome of disorders characterized by a distinctive, harsh, "barking" repetitive cough and hoarseness, resulting from inflammation in the area of the larynx. Croup syndromes may affect all areas of the upper respiratory system. Because the larynx is very small in infants and small children, inflammation may become obstructive.

ASL

Acute spasmodic laryngitis (ASL) occurs in children from 3 months to 3 years and usually appears suddenly at night with severe cough, dyspnea, and restlessness that awakens the child. Fever is absent. The symptoms usually are not evident in the daytime but do tend to recur. ASL may be related to allergies.

Treatment includes:

- Usually cool humidifiers are used in the child's room, but acute attacks may be relieved by the warm steam of hot running water (such as a running shower) in a closed room. Some children may stop coughing if exposed to cold air.
- Occasionally corticosteroids may be used to reduce inflammation.

Acute Epiglottitis

Acute epiglottitis (supraglottitis) occurs in children primarily from 1-8 years of age although it can occur at any age. It requires immediate medical attention as it can rapidly become obstructive. The onset is usually very sudden and often occurs during the night. The child may awaken suddenly with a fever, but usually does not have a cough. The **symptoms** include:

- *Tripod position*: Child sits upright, leaning forward with chin out, mouth open, and tongue protruding.
- *Agitation:* The child appears restless, tense, and agitated.
- *Drooling:* Excess secretions combined with pain or dysphagia and mouth open position cause drooling.
- *Voice*: No hoarseness, but voice sounds thick and "froglike."
- *Cyanosis*: Color is usually pale and sallow initially but may progress to frank cyanosis.
- *Throat*: On examination, the epiglottis appears bright red and swollen. NOTE: the child's throat should not be examined with a tongue blade unless intubation and tracheostomy equipment are immediately available as the examination can trigger obstruction.

Historically, most cases were viral, caused by *H. influenza,* type B, but infections can also be bacterial, with infections caused by *Streptococci* becoming more common. Acute epiglottitis has declined in children since the Hib vaccine was introduced, and is now more common in adults, but it can still occur in children.

Treatment*:* Because this condition can lead to acute respiratory failure and carries a risk of death, immediate treatment is necessary. Treatments include:

- Antibiotics for suspected bacterial infections or as indicated by epiglottal cultures.
- *Respiratory support*, which may require intubation or tracheostomy and mechanical ventilation (especially for viral infection). Intubation may be very difficult because of the excessive swelling, so immediate tracheostomy may be required.
- *Corticosteroids* are usually administered during intubation.

Swelling induced by bacteria usually recedes within 24 hours and returns to normal within 3 days.

Acute Laryngotracheobronchitis

Acute laryngotracheobronchitis occurs in children from 3 months to 8 years (usually <5). It is a viral infection, usually caused by the human parainfluenza viruses, types 1, 2, and 3 and accounts for about 75% of the total cases. It usually follows an upper respiratory infection that slowly encompasses the larynx, resulting in swelling of the mucosa and a progressive onset of low-grade fever with characteristic "croupy" cough. Swelling can cause respiratory obstruction, resulting in acute respiratory acidosis and respiratory failure.

Treatment includes:

- Cool humidified air is usually best, but some respond to a warm steamy atmosphere or cool outside air.
- Nebulized racemic epinephrine may be used in the hospital setting, but it is very short acting and can have a rebound effect, so children should not be treated in the ER and released.
- Oral and nebulized steroids (dexamethasone, budesonide) have been shown in recent studies to provide relief, and are safe to use in the home.
- Intubation and ventilation as needed.

Acute Tracheitis

Acute tracheitis occurs in children from 1 month to 6 years and is usually caused by *Staphylococcus aureus,* with an increase in community-acquired MRSA (CA-MRSA), although Group A β-hemolytic *Streptococci* and *H. Influenzae* and other organisms are implicated. This disorder may present with symptoms similar to acute laryngotracheobronchitis, but often fails to respond to the same treatment and can result in airway obstruction and respiratory arrest, so diagnosis and treatment are critical. This condition is usually preceded by an upper respiratory infection with croupy cough and strider as well as a high fever. One difference between this and other forms of croup is the production of copious amounts of thick, purulent tracheal exudate, which are implicated in dyspnea and obstruction.

Treatment includes:

- *Intubation and mechanical ventilation* to ensure patency of airway. Tracheostomy may be necessary in some cases.
- *Antibiotic therapy* should include vancomycin if there are signs of multi-organ failure or increased incidence of CA-MRSA.

Acute Abdominal Trauma

Acute abdominal trauma in children may be blunt (85%) or penetrating (15%). Blunt trauma from motor vehicle accidents, pedestrian injuries (running into traffic), lap belt injury, and sports injuries are common causes of abdominal injury. About 5% of abdominal injuries are related to child abuse, such as punching or kicking a child in the abdomen.

- *Blunt injuries* comprise crush (compression), shear (tearing), and burst (sudden increased pressure). Because the rib cage in a young child remains elastic, there may be major internal damage from blunt trauma without rib fractures.
- *Penetrating wounds,* on the other hand, may be related to accidental impaling but are almost always related to gunshot wounds (high energy) or knife assaults (low energy). Gunshot wounds tend to cause more extensive damage than stab wounds. Children's organs are larger in proportion to body size than those of adults, so they are more at risk from penetrating wounds.

Splenic Injuries

The **spleen** is the most frequently injured solid organ in blunt trauma in children. Injuries to the spleen are the most common because it's not well protected by the elastic rib cage and is very vascular. Symptoms may be very non-specific. Kehr sign (radiating pain in left shoulder) indicates intra-abdominal bleeding and Cullen sign (ecchymosis around umbilicus) indicate hemorrhage from ruptured spleen. Some may have right upper abdominal pain although diffuse abdominal pain

42

often occurs with blood loss, associated with hypotension. Splenic injuries are classified according to the degree of injury:

1. Tear in splenic capsules or hematoma.
2. Laceration of parenchyma (<3 cm).
3. Laceration of parenchyma (>3cm).
4. Multiple lacerations of parenchyma or burst-type injury.

Treatment may be supportive if injury is not severe; otherwise, suturing of spleen may be needed. Because children risk infection with splenectomy, every effort (bed rest, transfusion, reduced activity for at least 8 weeks) is done to avoid surgery because the spleen will often heal spontaneously.

Gastric and Intestinal Injuries

Gastric injuries in children may result in perforation, primarily at the greater curvature. The risk increases if children are injured with a full stomach after eating a meal and suffer a lap belt injury or fall over the handlebars of a bicycle. Perforation results in severe pain, rigid abdomen, and bloody nasogastric drainage with peritonitis developing within hours, so early diagnosis and surgical repair must be done. Intestinal injuries from blunt trauma are rare in children although contusions and rupture can occur from lap belt injuries. Indications of rupture often appear 24-48 hours when the child presents with symptoms of peritonitis, such as distention, abdominal pain, absent bowel sounds, leukocytosis, fever, dyspnea, nausea and vomiting. Prompt antibiotic therapy and surgical repair with peritoneal lavage must be done. The abdominal wound may be left open to heal by secondary intention.

Hepatic Injuries

Hepatic injury is the most common cause of death from abdominal trauma and is often associated with multiple organ damage, so symptoms may be non-specific. Automobile accidents cause most blunt trauma but accidents with mountain bikes account for increasing hematomas of the central area of the liver. Neonatal hepatic injuries are often misdiagnosed. Elevation in liver transaminase levels indicates damage that may require CT examination with double contrast. Liver injuries are classified according to the degree of injury:

1. Tears in capsule with hematoma.
2. Laceration(s) of parenchyma (<3 cm).
3. Laceration(s) of parenchyma (<3 cm).
4. Destruction of 25-75% of lobe from burst injury.
5. Destruction of >75% of lobe from burst injury.
6. Avulsion [tearing away].

Almost all hepatic injuries in children (97%) are treated conservatively, primarily because studies show that most hemorrhage stops prior to surgery. Injuries may take 3-12 months to heal with supportive treatment and close monitoring.

Pancreatic Injuries

Pancreatic injuries can result from motor vehicle or handlebar accidents or assault with impact the abdominal area although it is not a common injury. Penetrating injuries (gunshot wounds and stabbings) are more common. Because of the location of the pancreas, impact compresses it against the vertebral column. About 90% of children with pancreatic injury sustain other abdominal injuries as well, making diagnosis difficult. Symptoms may include diffuse abdominal or epigastric pain and well as vomiting of bile. Pancreatic injuries are classified according to degree of injury:

1. Contusion, laceration but ducts intact.
2. Distal transection or injury of parenchyma with ductal injury.
3. Proximal transection or injury of parenchyma with probable ductal injury.
4. Combined injury of pancreas and duodenum.

CT scans provide the best tool for diagnosis. Surgical exploration and repair of severe damage is the most common treatment. Pancreatitis and diabetes mellitus may be long-term sequelae.

Blunt and Penetrating Thoracic Injuries Causing Cardiac Trauma

Blunt trauma is most commonly implicated in thoracic injury in children, accounting for about 81%. Many of these children will have multiple system injuries as well.

- The majority of blunt trauma thoracic injuries are vehicle-related, where the child is a passenger involved in a vehicle accident or is struck by an automobile while a pedestrian or riding a bicycle. Many of the injuries are caused by failure to use protective devices, such as seat belts.
- Falls, while common, rarely involve major trauma.
- Child abuse can result in severe thoracic trauma.

Penetrating trauma is rare in small children but common in older adolescents:

- *Small children*: injuries related to accidents, such as with farm equipment or plate glass. Gunshot injuries are usually accidental.
- *Adolescents*: Injuries related to gunshot and stab wounds, which are the result of assault rather than accident.

Penetrating Cardiac Injuries

The incidence of **penetrating cardiac injuries** has been on the rise, primarily associated with gunshot injuries and stabbings. The extent of damage caused by a stab wound is often easier to assess than gunshot wounds, which may be multiple and often result in unpredictable and widespread damage not only to the heart but other structures. There are two primary complications:

- Exsanguination is frequently related to gunshot wounds, and prognosis is very poor.
- Cardiac tamponade (compression of the heart from bleeding into the pericardial sac) is more common with knife wounds, but prognosis is fairly good with surgical repair.

Mortality rates are very high in the first hour after a penetrating cardiac injury, so it is imperative the child be taken immediately to a trauma center rather than attempt to stabilize the child at the site.

Diagnosis is generally evident upon admission.

Treatment is prompt surgical repair.

Traumatic Injury to the Great Vessels

Traumatic **injuries to the great vessels** most commonly result from severe decelerating blunt force or penetrating injuries, with aortic trauma the most common. If the aorta is torn, it will result in almost instant death, but in some cases, there is an incomplete laceration to the intimal lining (innermost membrane) of the aorta, causing an aortic hematoma or bulging. This lining, the adventitia, is quite strong and often will contain the rupture long enough to allow surgical repair. Other vessels may be injured as well, so careful examination must be done.

Diagnosis is made initially with chest x-ray or CT, which may show widening of the mediastinum and a misshapen aorta. If there are indications of injury, an aortogram or a combination of CT and transesophageal echocardiogram may be used to verify the injury.

Treatment requires surgical repair to avoid eventual rupture, during which other vessels are examined for clotting or internal injuries.

Myocardial Contusion

Myocardial contusion can occur if a child sustains significant blunt impact to the thoracic area, resulting in anteroposterior compression that can cause direct injury to the heart or interfere with circulation, which can cause destruction of myocardial cells. Pulmonary injury or rib fractures increase the risk of myocardial contusion. Symptoms may include pain or shortness of breath, but because other injuries may be present, determining what relates to the heart can be difficult. Injury is most commonly indicated by arrhythmias, which tend to be self-limiting, but must be monitored.

Diagnosis is usually made by EKG to determine if there are arrhythmias. If the results of the EKG are normal, usually further tests are not warranted. If there are significant clinical signs of contusion, then an echocardiogram is indicated.

Treatment consists of close monitoring and medications as indicated to control arrhythmias.

Acute Tubular Necrosis

Acute tubular necrosis (ATN) occurs when a hypoxic condition causes renal ischemia that damages tubular cells of the glomeruli so they are unable to adequately filter the urine, leading to acute renal failure. Causes include hypotension, hyperbilirubinemia, sepsis, surgery (especially cardiac or vascular), and birth complications. ATN may result from nephrotoxic injury related to obstruction or drugs, such as chemotherapy, acyclovir, and antibiotics, such as sulfonamides and streptomycin. **Symptoms** may be non-specific initially and include life-threatening complications: * Lethargy. * Nausea and vomiting. * Hypovolemia with low cardiac output and generalized vasodilation. * Fluid and electrolyte imbalance leading to hypertension, CNS abnormalities, metabolic acidosis, arrhythmias, edema, and congestive heart failure. |* Uremia leading to destruction of platelets and bleeding, neurological deficits, and disseminated intravascular coagulopathy (DIC).

Treatment includes:

- Identifying and treating underlying cause.
- Supportive care. Loop diuretics (in some cases), such as Lasix®. Antibiotics for infection.
- Discontinuation of nephrotoxic agents.
- Kidney dialysis. Infections can include pericarditis and sepsis.

Renal Trauma

Most **renal trauma** in children is the result of blunt trauma associated with motor vehicle accidents, falls, sports injuries, and child abuse although gunshot wounds and stabbings also occur with increasing frequency. Various staging systems are used, but overall injuries are graded by severity:

1. Contusion of cortex with fracture (tear) of small confined area.
2. Major fracture with peri-renal hematoma and/or extravasation of urine.
3. Multiple fractures with extensive bleeding.
4. Severe vascular disruption decreasing perfusion of kidney.

Kidney injuries are often accompanied by other trauma (75%) so **symptoms** may be complex:

- Pain in abdominal or flank area.
- Hematuria. Abrasions or contusions in flank or abdominal area. Shock.

Delayed symptoms may occur:

- Hypertension.
- Hydronephrosis.

Treatment is usually non-operative if the child is hemodynamically stable, based on evaluation by CT, especially for blunt trauma. Gunshot wounds usually require surgical exploration:

- Bed rest.
- Monitoring of blood counts and vital signs.

Head Trauma

Head trauma can occur as the result of birth injury, but intentional or unintentional blunt or penetrating trauma is usually caused by falls, automobile accidents, sports injuries, or child abuse. Head injury is the most common cause of death in children. The degree of injury correlates with the impact force. The skull of infants and young children is pliable and absorbs much impact, but a severe blow can cause significant neurological damage.

- *Acceleration-deceleration injuries* are those in which a blow to the stationary head causes the elastic skull to change shape, pushing against the brain, which moves sharply backward in response, striking against the skull.
- Bruising can occur at the point of impact (*coup*) and the point where the brain hits the skull (*contrecoup*). So a blow to the frontal area can cause damage to the occipital region.
- The sudden movement of the brain may cause *shear injuries*, where vessels are torn.
- *Severe compression* may force the brain through the tentorial opening, damaging the brainstem.

Complications

Concussions, Contusions, and Lacerations

A variety of different injuries can occur as a result of **head trauma**:

- *Concussions* are the most common injury and are usually relatively transient, causing no permanent neurological damage. They may result in confusion, disorientation, and mild amnesia, but last only minutes or hours.
- *Contusions/lacerations* are bruising and tears of cerebral tissue. There may be petechial areas at the impact site (coup) or larger bruising. Contrecoup injuries are less common in children than in adults. Areas most impacted by contusions and lacerations are the occipital, frontal, and temporal lobes. The degree of injury relates to the amount of vascular damage, but initial symptoms are similar to concussion; however, symptoms persist and may progress, depending upon the degree of injury. Lacerations are often caused by fractures. Because of the extensive vascularity of a child's scalp, large scalp lacerations related to head injuries can result in major hemorrhage.

Cerebral Edema and Increased Intracranial Pressure

Head injuries that occur at the time of trauma include fractures, contusions, hematomas, and diffuse cerebral and vascular injury. These injuries may result in hypoxia, increased intracranial pressure, and cerebral edema. Open injuries may result in infection. Often the primary problem with head trauma in children is a significant increase in swelling, which interferes with perfusion, causing hypoxia and hypercapnia, which trigger increased blood flow. This increased volume at a time when injury impairs auto-regulation increases cerebral edema, which, in turn, increases intracranial pressure and results in a further decrease in perfusion with ischemia. If pressure continues to rise, the brain may herniate. Concomitant hypotension may result in hypoventilation, further complicating treatment. Children seem to tolerate this increase in pressure better than adults, perhaps because the skull is pliable and allows for some expansion. However, while children often have smaller lesions after trauma than adults, they may have more long-term sequelae.

Fractures

Fractures are a common cause of penetrating wounds causing cerebral lacerations. Much force is needed to fracture the flexible skull of a small child; however, meningeal arteries lie in groves on the underside of the skull, and a fracture can cause an arterial tear and hemorrhage. Skull fractures include:

- *Basilar:* Occurs in bones at the base of the brain and can cause severe brainstem damage.
- *Comminuted:* Skull fractures into small pieces.
- *Compound:* Surface laceration extends to a skull fracture.
- *Depressed:* Pieces of the skull are depressed inward on the brain tissue, often producing dural tears, usually occurring in children >2-3 years when the skull is less elastic.
- *Diastatic:* Causes separation of the skull along cranial sutures, most commonly the lambdoid suture, usually ≥ 4 years. Typically caused by impact with large flat surface, such as a wall.
- *Linear:* Impact causes a depression and a buckling outward of the surrounding skull, usually >2-3 years.

Shaken Baby/Shaken Impact Syndrome

Shaken baby syndrome is believed to be the result of vigorous shaking of an infant, causing acute subdural hematoma with subarachnoid and retinal hemorrhages. It is believed that the shaking of the brain causes both coup and contrecoup damage as well as damaging vessels and nerves with resultant cerebral edema. Some authorities, however, believe that the extent of injuries typically seen with these infants precludes just shaking and that they must also suffer blunt impact, as the injuries are more compatible with the head striking against a solid surface with great force, so the newer terminology is **shaken impact syndrome**, which includes shaking AND impact. **Symptoms** include:

- Mortality rate of about 50%.
- Severe residual problems that may include vision and hearing defects, seizures, intellectual disability or impaired cognition, paralysis, or coma.

Sometimes children may not exhibit obvious neurological symptoms immediately after trauma but have learning disabilities and behavioral disorders that appear in school.

Intracranial/Intraventricular Hemorrhage

Epidural

Hemorrhage is always a concern with head trauma because even injuries that appear slight can result in vascular rupture, resulting in hemorrhage between the skull and the brain. There are two types of hemorrhage that often occur from head trauma: epidural and subdural. **Epidural hemorrhage** is bleeding between the dura and the skull, pushing the brain downward and inward. The hemorrhage is usually caused by arterial tears, so bleeding is often rapid, leading to severe neurological deficits and respiratory arrest. Initially, the body compensates by rapidly absorbing cerebrospinal fluid and decreasing blood flow, but the compensatory measure is soon overwhelmed. The most common site is the parietotemporal region, forcing the medial part of the temporal lobe under the tentorial edge, compressing nerves and vessels. This type of injury usually results from unintentional falls and rarely from child abuse. It is not common in children <4 years. Diagnosis in small children is often delayed because of nonspecific symptoms.

Subdural

Subdural hemorrhage is bleeding between the dura and the cerebrum, usually from tears in the cortical veins of the subdural space. It tends to develop more slowly than epidural hemorrhage and can result in a subdural hematoma. If the bleeding is acute and develops within minutes or hours of injury, the prognosis is poor. Subacute hematomas that develop more slowly cause varying degrees of injury. Subdural hemorrhage is a common injury related to birth trauma but is otherwise usually caused by child abuse, although it can result from coagulopathies or aneurysms. **Symptoms** of acute injury may occur within 24-48 hours, but subacute bleeding may not be evident for up to 2 weeks after injury. Chronic hemorrhage occurs primarily in the elderly. Symptoms vary and may include bradycardia, tachycardia, hypertension, and alterations in consciousness. Subdural taps may suffice for infants, but some infants and older children will require surgical evacuation of the hematoma.

Subarachnoid

Subarachnoid hemorrhage is a common injury after trauma and may result from the childbirth (one of the most common causes) or from abuse (shaken impact syndrome) along with subdural hematoma. While less common in children than adults, subarachnoid hemorrhage can also occur from rupture of a berry aneurysm or an arteriovenous malformation (AVM). However, there are a number of disorders that may be implicated: neoplasms, sickle cell disease, infection, hemophilia, and leukemia. The first presenting symptom in infants may be seizures, and usually symptoms are similar to those of subdural hematoma. Older children may complain of severe headache, nausea

48

and vomiting, nuchal rigidity, palsy related to cranial nerve compression, retinal hemorrhages, and papilledema. Symptoms will worsen as intracranial pressure rises. **Treatment** includes:

- Identifying and treating underlying cause.
- Anti-seizure medications (such as Dilantin®) to control seizures.
- Antihypertensives.
- Surgical repair if indicated.

Symptoms of Increased Intracranial Pressure

Because the brain in the skull has limited expansion room, any increase in the volume of one component (brain, cerebrospinal fluid, or blood) must be compensated for with a decrease in another component to keep volume and pressure balanced. Children have open fontanels that allow for some expansion; however, the ability to compensate is limited, and trauma, tumors, bleeding, fluid accumulation in the ventricles, or edema of the tissues can cause **increased intracranial pressure**. Symptoms may vary with age:

- *Infants*: Bulging fontanels without normal pulsations, distention of scalp veins, and increased head circumference. Infants may be irritable with high-pitched cries and poor feeding.
- *Children*: Headache, vomiting without associated nausea, double and blurred vision, seizures. Behavioral and personality changes may occur, increased lethargy, memory loss, and inability to follow directions.
- *Late signs:* Decreased level of consciousness, motor response, and response to painful stimuli. Pupil size and reactivity changes decerebrate or decorticate posturing, respiratory depression with Cheyne-Stokes may occur as well as papilledema.

Symptoms of Acute Brain Injury

Infants and small children often exhibit symptoms of **acute brain injury** that are non-specific or different than the typical symptoms of adults. There may be associated injuries, such as laceration or bruising evident:

- *Mild injuries:* Children may be irritable and restless or somnolent and listless. They may lose consciousness or have periods of confusion. Pallor and vomiting are common.
- *Progressive injuries:* As the condition worsens, alterations of consciousness appear, and children may be difficult to rouse. There may be agitation and marked fluctuations in vital signs, as well as focal neurological deficits (paralysis, spasticity, paresis, or lack of sensation in one part of the body).
- *Severe injuries:* Children may show signs of increased intracranial pressure, retinal hemorrhage, hemiparesis/hemiplegia or quadriparesis/quadriplegia, thermal deregulation with elevated temperature. Older children may exhibit uncoordinated gait and papilledema.

Childhood Strokes

Strokes (brain attacks) can occur in infants and children and may result from ischemic disruption of blood flow or hemorrhage. Onset may be quite sudden. Neonate may present with hypotonia, seizure, and respiratory distress while older children may have symptoms that include sudden headache, weakness, numbness, hemiplegia, confusion, vision disturbances, dysphagia, poor feeding, and difficulty speaking, depending upon the site and extent of the stroke. They occur as a result of a number of disorders:

- Autoimmune disorders, such as antiphospholipid antibody syndrome.
- Congenital disorders, such as arteriovenous malformation, congenital heart disease, and sickle cell.
- Birth trauma.
- Clotting disorders.
- Disseminated intravascular coagulopathy (DIC).
- Toxins (cocaine, amphetamines).
- Embolus.
- Moyamoya.
- Head trauma.
- Surgery.
- Chemotherapy (especially with asparaginase).
- Infections such as chicken pox, encephalitis, meningitis, and HIV.

Residual effects may include cerebral palsy, seizure disorders, hemiparesis/hemiplegia, hypotonia or spasticity, speech impairment, and vision impairment.

Treatment Options

While some authorities recommend **stroke treatment** for infants and children similar to that of adults, for both immediate treatment and preventive measures, such as tPA (tissue plasminogen activator) and anticoagulation therapy, studies indicate that diagnosis is often delayed more than 24 hours, precluding treatment, such as tPA that should be initiated within 3-6 hours of onset of symptoms. Some studies have indicated that children receiving tPA often are given delayed treatments. Further, even though children often have recurrent strokes, preventive therapy, such as anticoagulation, is often not instituted. Adequate studies showing the efficacy of these therapies and proper dosages are limited, making therapeutic decisions difficult for physicians; however, use of tPA has increased because the outlook for children with strokes is grim. Strokes in children have a 10% mortality rate and 60% residual disability rate. Thus, much treatment is aimed at controlling symptoms, such as seizures, and rehabilitation through physical therapy, aquatic therapy, and speech therapy.

Anaphylaxis Syndrome

Anaphylaxis syndrome is a sudden acute systemic immunoglobulin E (IgE) or non-immunoglobulin E (non-IgE) inflammatory response affecting the cardiopulmonary and other systems.

- *IgE-mediated response* (anaphylactic shock) is an antibody-antigen reaction against an allergen, such as milk, peanuts, latex, insect bites, or fish. This is the most common type.
- *Non IgE-mediated response* (anaphylactoid reaction) is a systemic reaction to infection, exercise, radio contrast material or other triggers. While the response is almost identical to the other type, it does not involve IgE.

Typically, with IgE-mediated response, an antigen triggers release of substances, such as histamine and prostaglandins, which affect the skin, cardiopulmonary, and GI systems. Histamine causes initial erythema and edema by inducing vasodilation. Each time the child has contact with the antigen, more antibodies form in response, so allergic reactions worsen with each contact. In some cases, initial reactions may be mild, but subsequent contact can cause severe life-threatening response.

Symptoms and Treatment

Anaphylaxis syndrome may present with a few symptoms or a wide range that encompasses cardiopulmonary, dermatological, and gastrointestinal responses. **Symptoms** may recur after the initial treatment (biphasic anaphylaxis) in about 6% of children, so careful monitoring is essential:

- Sudden onset of weakness, dizziness, confusion.
- Severe generalized edema and angioedema. Lips and tongue may swell. Urticaria.
- Increased permeability of vascular system and loss of vascular tone. Severe hypotension leading to shock.
- Laryngospasm/bronchospasm with obstruction of airway causing dyspnea and wheezing. Nausea, vomiting, and diarrhea. Seizures, coma and death.

Treatment includes:

- Establish patent airway and intubate if necessary.
- Provide oxygen at 100% high flow.
- Monitor VS.
- Administer epinephrine (Epi-pen® or 1:1000 solution t 0.1mg/kg/wt).
- 2.5mg albuterol per nebulizer for *bronchospasm*. Intravenous fluids to provide bolus of fluids for *hypotension*. Diphenhydramine 1.0 mg/kg/wt (to 25 mg) if *shock* persists. Methylprednisolone 2.0 mg/kg/wt if no response to other drugs.

Injury Prevention

Environmental Assessment

Environmental Factors

Environmental factors should be assessed within the **actual environment** if at all possible. If not, careful questioning and drawing of diagrams and approximate floor plans with the patient—or asking the patient to do drawings—can be useful, especially when showing the patient needed modifications. Family members may also assist with the assessment, providing useful information. Some patients, especially the elderly, may be reluctant to admit that the home is cluttered or that they are unable to maintain the home environment in a sanitary condition. Brochures and handouts about home safety and assistive devices should be provided to the patient as well as contact names and numbers for equipment needed in the home. A checklist should be compiled of all necessary changes or additions, with specific details, such as "Install 18-inch grab bar across from toilet." In some cases, a social worker or occupational therapist should visit the patient.

General Elements of Assessment

Some elements of an **environmental assessment** are not specific to rooms in the house but are general needs that must be met in order for people, especially the elderly or disabled, to remain safe:

- **Environmental hazards** such as piles of papers or junk on the floors, loose carpet or rugs, and cluttered pathways can cause falls and must be cleared, organized, or repaired.
- **Lighting** should be adequate enough for reading in all rooms and stairways.

- **Heat and air conditioning** must be adequate. The young and the elderly are especially susceptible to heat and cold injury.
- **Sanitation** should ensure that health hazards do not exist, such as from rotting food or infestations of cockroaches or rodents.
- **Animals** should be cared for adequately with access to food, water, toileting, and routine veterinary care.
- **Smoke/chemicals** in the environment may pose a hazard, such as exposure to cigarette smoking or cleaning materials.

Disaster Management Plans

There are several different types of **disaster management plans**, some more specific than others. They are listed and briefly described below:

- **Emergency Action Plan** – OSHA required, evacuation plans and emergency drills.
- **Business Continuity Plan** – Business operation-specific, aimed at reducing losses and resuming productivity.
- **Risk Management Plan** – Off-site effects of chemical exposures.
- **Emergency Response Plan** – Immediate response to disasters.
- **Contingency Plan** – General, designed to handle events not covered in other plans.
- **Federal Response Plan** – Coordinates federal resources.
- **Spill Prevention, Control, and Countermeasures Plan** – Deals with the prevention, control, and clean-up of oil spills.
- **Mutual Aid Plan** – Plan for shared resources between other companies/firms.
- **Recovery Plan** – Deals with repair and rebuilding post-disaster.
- **Emergency Management Plan** – Plan for healthcare facilities.
- **All-Hazard Disaster Management Plan** – General plan that is not hazard-specific.

Development

There are many different types of **disaster management plans**. Regardless of the type, however, there are several basic steps for its development. To begin with, a **planning team** must be established that includes representatives from all levels within the organization. The planning team is responsible for putting together a timeline for completion of the plan as well as an estimation of the costs, fees, and resources necessary to complete the plan. Once this is done, an **analysis of potential disasters** can begin. In this step, potential hazards are identified and vulnerability of the organization to disasters is assessed. A disaster response plan is established that includes the reduction/removal of hazardous situations. The final steps are **plan implementation and review**. The plan can be tested for efficacy through drills and mock disaster situations. It is critical to review and update the plan yearly.

Environmental Emergencies

Rape and Sexual Abuse

Rape and sexual abuse victims (both male and female) should be treated sensitively and questioned privately. Examination should include:

- **Assault history** that includes what happened, when, where, and by whom. Questioning should determine if there is a possibility of drug-induced amnesia or activities, such as douching or showering, which might have destroyed evidence.

- **Medical history** to determine if there is a risk of pregnancy and when and if the last consensual sex occurred that might interfere with laboratory findings.
- **Physical examination** should include examination of the genitals, rectum, and mouth. The body should be examined for bruising or other injuries. Toluidine dye should be applied to the perineum before insertion of a speculum into the vagina to detect small vulvar lacerations.

Forensic evidence must be collected within 72 hours and requires informed consent and the use of a rape kit. Forensic evidence includes:

- Victim samples for control.
- Assailant-identifying samples
- Evidence of sexual activity.
- Evidence of force or coercion.

Animal Bites

There is no one typical therapy for **traumatic wounds** because they vary so widely in the type and degree of injury. A cat scratch on the knee is treated very differently from a shark attack that involves massive tissue injury or tissue loss. Animal bites, including human, are frequent causes of traumatic injury. Treatment includes:

- **Cleanse** wound by flushing with 10-35 cc syringe with 18-gauge Angiocath to remove debris and bacteria using normal saline or dilute Betadine® solution.
- Hand, puncture, and infected wounds or those more than 12 hours old may be closed by **secondary intention**.
- **Moisture-retentive dressings** as indicated by the size and extent of injury of wound left open. **Dry dressings** may be applied to injuries with closure by primary intention.
- **Topical antibiotics** may be indicated although systemic antibiotics are commonly prescribed for animal bites.
- Tetanus toxoid or immune globulin is routinely administered.

Tick Bites

Ticks, blood-feeding parasites, are the primary vector of infectious diseases in the United States. Ticks transmit a wide variety of **pathogens**, including bacteria such as Rickettsiae, protozoan parasites, and viruses. **Lyme disease** is the most common tick-borne disease, but there are increasing reports of other diseases, such as babesiosis, human anaplasmosis, and ehrlichiosis. Many tick-borne diseases present with similar non-specific flu-like symptoms and can easily be misdiagnosed. Ticks should be carefully removed if still feeding:

- Using fine-tipped **tweezers**, tick is grasped close to the skin and pulled upward with even and steady pressure, avoiding jerks or twists that may break mouthparts.
- The tick must not be handled with **bare hands**.
- **Disinfect** skin site.
- Tick should be saved for **identification**: place tick in a plastic bag, date, and place in freezer in case illness occurs in 2 to 3 weeks.

People should be cautioned to immediately seek medical attention for **flu-like or neurological symptoms** or **erythema migrans** (bullseye rash) typical of Lyme disease.

Bee Stings

Bees and wasps sting by puncturing the skin with a hollow stinger and injecting **venom**. Wasps and bumblebees can sting more than once but honeybees have barbs on their stingers, and the barbs keep the stinger hooked into the skin. Local reactions to bee sting:

- Raised white **weal** with central red spot of about 10 mm appearing within a few minutes and lasting 20 minutes (honeybees)
- **Edema and erythema**, which may last several days (Vespid wasps).
- Pain, swelling, and redness confined to **sting site**.
- Swelling may extend **beyond the sting site** and may, for example involve swelling of an entire limb.

Some people may develop an **anaphylactic reaction**, including a biphasic reaction, in which the symptoms recede and then return 2-3 hours later. About 50% of deaths occur within 30 minutes of the sting, and 75% within 4 hours. Symptoms of an allergic reaction/anaphylaxis may become increasingly severe with generalized urticaria, edema, hypotension, and respiratory distress.

Treatment of **bee stings** initially includes:

- **Wash** the site with soap and water.
- **Remove** stinger using a 4x4-inch gauze wiped over the area or by scraping a sharp instrument over the area.
- NEVER **squeeze** the stinger or use tweezers, as this will cause more venom to go into the skin.
- Apply **ice** to reduce the swelling (10-20 minutes on/10-20 minutes off for 24 hours).
- **Antihistamines** may be prescribed.
- A paste of **baking soda and water** or meat tenderizer and water may reduce itching.
- **Topical corticosteroids** may relieve itching.
- Tetanus toxoid or tetanus immune globulin as needed.

Allergic responses/anaphylaxis require **immediate aggressive medical intervention**: Epinephrine, antihistamines, corticosteroids, oxygen and other supportive treatment, and IV fluids as needed. People with extensive local or anaphylactic reactions should be advised to carry an EpiPen® for emergency use if stung.

Spider Bites

Spider bites are frequently a misdiagnosis of a Staphylococcus aureus or methicillin-resistant Staphylococcus aureus (MRSA) infection, so unless the spider was observed, the wound should be cultured and antibiotics started. If the wound responds to the antibiotic, then it probably wasn't a spider bite. There are 2 main types of venomous spider bites:

- Producing **neurological symptoms** (Black widow).
- Producing **local necrosis** (brown recluse, yellow sac, and hobo spiders).

Treatment includes:

- Cleanse wound and apply cool compress and elevate body part if possible.
- Black widow bites:
  - Narcotic analgesics.
  - Nitroprusside to relieve hypertension.
  - Calcium gluconate 10% solution IV for abdominal cramps.
  - Latrodectus antivenin for those with severe reaction.
- Necrotic/ulcerated bites (brown recluse, etc.).
  - There is no consensus on the best treatment as ulceration caused by the venom may be extensive and surgical repair with grafts may be needed.
  - Treatment as for other necrotic ulcers, with moisture retentive dressings as indicated.
  - Hyperbaric oxygen therapy (HBOT) used in some cases.

Snake Bites

About 45,000 **snake bites** occur in the United States each year, with about 8000 poisonous. In the United States, about 25 species of snakes are venomous. There are 2 types of snakes that can cause serious injury, classified according to the type of fangs and venom.

Coral Snakes

Coral snakes have short fixed permanent fangs in the upper jaw and venom that is primarily neurotoxic, but may also have hemotoxic and cardiotoxic properties:

- Wounds show no fang marks but there may be scratches or semi-circular markings from teeth.
- There may be little local reaction, but neurological symptoms may range from mild to acute respiratory and cardiovascular failure.

Treatment includes:

- Cleansing wound thoroughly of dirt and debris and leave open or cover with dry dressing.
- Antibiotics not usually needed.
- Administering antivenin immediately even without symptoms, which may be delayed.
- Tetanus toxoid or immune globulin.

Pit Vipers

A second type that can cause serious injury are the **pit vipers. Rattlesnakes, copperheads, and cottonmouths** have erectile fangs that fold until they are aroused, and venom is primarily hemotoxic and cytotoxic but may have neurotoxic properties.

- Wounds usually show 1-2 fang marks.
- Edema may begin immediately or may be delayed up to 6 hours.
- Pain may be severe.
- There may be a wide range of symptoms, including hypotension and coagulopathy with defibrination that can lead to excessive blood loss, depending upon the type and amount of venom.
- There may be local infection and necrosis.

Treatment includes:

- Cleansing wound thoroughly and dressings as indicated.
- Tetanus toxoid or immune globulin.
- Analgesics, such as morphine sulphate
- Avoiding NSAIDs and aspirin because of anticoagulation properties.
- Marking edema every 15 minutes.
- Antivenin therapy if indicated (observation for serum sickness if horse serum used).
- Prophylactic antibiotics for severe tissue necrosis.
- Platelets, plasma, or packed RBCs for coagulopathy.

Dangerous Weapons and Toys

Parents should be advised to avoid keeping **guns** in the home or to keep guns unloaded and locked in a secure cabinet or container with the ammunition locked away in a different area from the gun. All children, from an early age, should be taught to never pick up a gun or point it at anyone, even in play, and to immediately tell a trusted adult if they see anyone with a gun or know of anyone, such as a peer, who is carrying a gun or intends to harm someone with a gun.

Children should be protected from **dangerous toys**, which can include toys with small parts that may cause choking, especially for infants and toddlers. Toys that shoot projectiles, have cords or strings attached, or have sharp edges may pose a risk as well. Some products, such as some types of slime, have been found to contain toxins, so parents should regularly check with the U.S. Consumer Product Safety Commission for alerts and should always read and adhere to warning labels. Smart toys and electronic devices that connect to the Internet may provide identifying information about the child to unauthorized individuals.

Children Presenting with Toxic Ingestions

Assessment

Pediatric poisoning is one of the most common medical problems with young children, accounting for about 5% of childhood mortality. Over 90% of poisonings occur within the home environment and over half of toxic poisonings occur to children <6. Most poisonings of young children are accidental and involve small amounts of one substance, generally a household product, such as cosmetics, or medications. Adolescent poisoning is more often intentional, as a suicide attempt or substance abuse, often with multiple substances ingested and a delay in treatment. Recreational drugs, such as Ecstasy, have been implicated in increased poisonings. Assessment of children with suspected ingestion of toxic substances includes:

- **A**irway. **B**reathing. **C**irculation.
- **D**isability, drugs/decontamination **E**CG, exposure.

Thorough examination to determine the *toxidrome* (characteristic patterns of *symptoms* related to specific toxins) must include assessment of the following:

- Vital sign changes.
- Alterations in mental status.
- Specific symptoms.
- Clinical findings.
- Results of laboratory testing, including serum and urine toxicology screens.

<u>Treatment</u>

Treatment for **toxic ingestions** is related to the type of toxin and whether or not it is identified. **Treatment** includes:

- *Administering antidote* if substance is known and an antidote exists. Antidotes for common toxins include:
    - Opiates: Naloxone (Narcan®)
    - Toxic alcohols: Ethanol infusion and/or dialysis.
    - Acetaminophen: N-acetylcysteine.
    - Calcium channel blockers, beta-blockers:
        - ❖ Calcium chloride
        - ❖ Glucagon
    - Tricyclic antidepressants: Sodium bicarbonate.
- *GI decontamination*- at one time this was a standard procedure (Ipecac® and gastric lavage followed by activated charcoal), but it is no longer advised for routine use, although selective gastric lavage may be appropriate if done within 1 hour of ingestion.
- *Activated charcoal* (1 g/kg/wt) orally or per NG tube binds to many toxins if given within one hour of ingestion. It may also be used in multiple doses (q 4-6 hrs) to enhance elimination.
- *Forced diuresis* with alkalization of urine (>7.5) may prevent absorption of drugs that are weak bases or acids.

Recommendations for Parents and Children Regarding Social Situations

<u>Strangers and Violence</u>

Recommendations for **social situations** include:

- *Strangers*: Parents should stress the importance of going places and playing outside with a friend or an adult and avoiding being alone. Children should be aware to run and yell if a stranger asks them to carry something, help get something out of a car, or to help look for or see a puppy or kitten. Parents should stress that children should never get into a car with a stranger or acquaintance who says that the child's parent has sent the person unless this person uses a password. Children should know to yell what is happening ("This woman is taking me!") and should know their full name, address, and phone number as soon as they are old enough to learn them.
- *Violence*: Parents should limit children's exposure to violent media content (TV, movies, video games) and use blocking tools when appropriate. Parents should encourage children to talk about their feeling if they've experienced or observed violence and to reassure them. If violence is common, children should play only in safe areas and learn safety rules, such as dropping to the ground if they hear gunshots.

<u>Bullying and Automobile Safety/Distracted Driving</u>

Recommendations for **social situations** include:

- *Bullying*: Parents should recognize the signs that a child is being bullied (depression, withdrawal, dislike of school, change in affect, lack of friends, change of sleep patterns, bruises) and teach children the impact that bullying has on others. Advise parents to tell children to tell an adult if they are being bullied and to respond assertively, to act unimpressed, to make a joke out of mean comments, and to get involved in activities, such as clubs, where they feel safe. If cyberbullied, they should block the senders, change passwords, and report it to an adult.
- *Automobile safety/Distracted driving*: Children should be seated and secured properly for their age and size and should be taught to avoid yelling, throwing things, and scuffling while in the car as this may distract the driver. Teenage drivers should be taught safe driving (including never driving while drinking), should have clear consequences for unsafe driving (such as loss of driving privileges), and should have an app on phones that prevents texting while driving and provides location.

Recommendations Regarding Sports and Recreation

<u>Concussions</u>

Recommendations regarding **sports and recreation** include:

- *Concussion risks*: Greatest risks are from sports activities (football, hockey, soccer, lacrosse) and accidents (fall, car/bicycle). Parents should ensure that any sports team a child participates in has adequate safety rules (limits to tackling, for example) and that coaches carefully monitor the children. Children should always wear appropriate safety gear, such as helmets, when engaged in sports activities and should never continue playing if exhibiting any signs of head injury (headache, dizziness, confusion).
- *Helmet use*: Helmets (the appropriate type) should be worn for sports activities that may involve falls or blows to the head (hockey, football, skateboarding, baseball, bicycling). Helmets should fit snuggly so that they don't move if they are rotated, turned, or tilted, and the helmet should be pressed down at the crown to check for fitting of the jaw pads and chin straps. Football helmets may be air/fluid filled or padded.

<u>Drowning Accidents</u>

Drowning is the leading cause of death in children <5 and the second in children <15:

- *Infants:* Bathtub injuries usually associated with intentional injury or lack of supervision.
- *Toddler:* Injuries in pools, bathtub, spa, toilet, places where children have access with lack of supervision.
- *Children:* Injuries in swimming pool or spa.
- *Adolescents:* Injuries in lakes, rivers, oceans related to risk-taking, altered level of awareness because of drugs or alcohol.

Submersion usually causes aspiration (wet drowning) but may trigger severe laryngospasm (dry drowning):

- Laryngospasm leads to this sequence:
    o Cardiac arrest with hypoxia/acidosis to brain.
    o Decreased oxygen, glucose, and adenosine triphosphate.

- o Decreased sodium, potassium pump.
- o Increased Na and water in ICF.
- o Cerebral intracellular edema leading to neuronal death.
- Aspiration leads to this sequence:
  - o Cardiac arrest with hypoxic/acidosis to other organs (heart, kidneys). Decreased oxygen, glucose, adenosine triphosphate.
  - o Decreased sodium, potassium pump. Increased Na and water in ICF. Hypovolemia with shock and death.

Near-Drowning Asphyxia

Submersion asphyxiation can cause profound damage to the central nervous system, pulmonary dysfunction related to aspiration, cardiac hypoxia with life-threatening arrhythmias, fluid and electrolyte imbalances, and multi-organ damage, so treatment can be complex. Hypothermia related to near drowning has some protective affect because blood is shunted to the brain and heart. *Treatment* includes:

- Immediate establishment of airway, breathing and circulation (ABCs).
- High flow 100% oxygen with face mask or intubation if respiratory distress worsens.
- NG tube and decompression to reduce risk of aspiration.
- Fluid management to prevent/ control cerebral/pulmonary edema.
- Neurological evaluation.
- Pulmonary management includes monitoring for ≥72 hours for respiratory deterioration. Ventilation may need positive-end expiratory pressure (PEEP), but this poses danger to cardiac output and can cause barotrauma, so use should be limited.
- Monitoring of cardiac output and function.
- Neurological care to reduce cerebral edema and increased intracranial pressure, and prevent secondary injury.
- Treat GI stress ulcers and acute renal failure.

Vehicle Safety

Boat Safety

According to U.S. Coast Guard's recommendations for **boat safety**, infants who are not of the appropriate weight and size to wear approved personal flotation devices (PFDs) should not be taken on recreational boats (rowboats, motorboats, kayaks, sailboats). All other children should wear life jackets that are properly fitted and secured. PFDs do not include swimming aids intended for play, such as water wings or pool noodles. If an infant is on a boat, a caregiver wearing a life jacket should hold the infant at all times and should not place the child in a car seat (which will not float). Infants and young children are more likely to develop hypothermia, so they should be wrapped with a dry blanket or towel if cold and shivering. Children by about age 3 should be taught safety rules, such as keeping hands and feet inside the boat and walking instead of running. All children should take swimming lessons. Older children should take a boat safety course if possible. Adolescents, especially, should be cautioned to never engage in drinking or recreational drug use while boating.

Car Seats

All infants, regardless of age, must be placed properly in an **infant car seat** during transit. Holding an infant while the car is in motion is not safe. Car seats should be new or in very good condition and fastened according to manufacturer's guidelines to ensure safety:

- Place the car seat in the back seat and away from any side airbags.
- Always securely buckle the child into the seat.
- Face the infant seat toward the rear of the car.
- Recline the seat so that the infant's head does not fall forward.
- Place padding around (not under) the infant if the infant slouches to one side.
- Place blankets OVER the straps and buckles, not under.

The infant/toddler should be placed in the rear-facing seat to the maximum weight and height allowed by the seat (some accommodate up to 65 pounds). Once transitioned to front-facing seats, children should be placed in belt-positioning booster seats until the vehicle's seat/shoulder belts fit properly (usually until 4' 9" and 8-12 years old). Until age 13, children should sit secured in the back seat and not the front.

Risk Taking Behaviors

Leading Causes of Death in the Birth to 10-Year Age Group

For the **birth to 10-year** age group, the US Preventive Services Task Force has assembled a list of the **5 leading causes of death**. The number 1 cause of death in this age group is actually a group of conditions that arise in the time period surrounding birth (the "**perinatal period**"). There are a number of conditions that arise surrounding birth that are fatal, including placental problems (premature separation, abruption), umbilical cord problems (cord prolapse, nuchal cord, single umbilical artery), infections (chorioamnionitis, congenital pneumonia), trauma during the birthing process (nerve damage, intracranial hemorrhage), and hemolytic disease of the newborn. The second leading cause of death is attributed to **congenital defects**, including tetralogy of Fallot, transposition of the great arteries, spina bifida, and anencephaly. Other leading causes of death include **sudden infant death syndrome (SIDS), motor vehicle injuries, and other unintentional injuries**.

Injury Prevention in Birth to 10-Year Age Group

Injury prevention counseling is a strong recommendation for the **birth to 10-year** age group, owing to the fact that motor vehicle accidents and other unintentional accidents are leading causes of death for this population. Children (and their parents) should be advised to use car safety seats until the age of 5 (this is subject to state law, however, as some states require the use of booster seats until a certain height or age is reached). After the age of 5, standard safety belts should always be used. When biking, skating, or skateboarding, a helmet should always be worn; these activities should not take place in the street. Parents should be advised to become CPR certified. They should also be advised to keep drugs, poisons, guns and other weapons, and matches out of the reach of children; to install smoke detectors and plan an escape route in the event of fire; and to make sure that stairs, windows, and pools are safe for children.

Leading Causes of Death in 11 to 24-Year Age Population

The list of the top 5 leading causes of death in the **11-24** age population differs significantly from the leading causes of death in the birth to 10-year age population. Leading the list for age 11-24 are deaths caused by either **motor vehicle accidents or other unintentional accidents**. Second on the list is **homicide**, followed by **suicide** as the third leading cause of death. The fourth leading cause of death in the 11-24 age population is **cancer**; the most common fatal cancers in this age group include leukemia (acute lymphocytic leukemia and acute myeloid leukemia), brain tumors (medulloblastoma, astrocytoma, and brainstem glioma), rhabdomyosarcoma, neuroblastoma, Wilms tumor, Ewing sarcoma, and Hodgkin lymphoma. The fifth leading cause of death in this age population is due to **general heart diseases**, which may include cardiomyopathies and faulty valves.

Youth Risk Surveillance System

The **Youth Risk Surveillance System** (YRSS) is a program conducted through the CDC that monitors six different categories of health-risk behaviors of adolescents:

- Behaviors relating to injuries and violence.
- Tobacco use.
- Alcohol and other drug use.
- High-risk sexual behavior that can result in unwanted pregnancy and sexually-transmitted diseases, including HIV.
- Nutrition.
- Exercise.

The YRSS gathers data from 40 states and 21 local surveys (such as large cities) from grades 9-12 and then compiles the information, assessing for trends. Responses are either weighted (≥60% participation) or unweighted (relates only to those completing survey). Weighted results can be generalized to the teenage population at large in the area of the survey. Information is also gathered about obesity and asthma in teenagers. The data obtained in the YRSS is used to determine progress in 15 national health objectives for health promotion.

Health-Risk Behaviors

Tobacco Use

The CDC conducts the Youth Risk Surveillance System to determine health-risk behaviors that contribute to significant morbidity in adolescents. **Tobacco,** often thought of as an adult issue, is a cause of concern for children and teenagers. Tobacco use is one of the leading preventable causes of death in the United States, but about 70% of children have tried smoking before high school, often beginning by age 12, putting themselves at risk for heart and lung disease as adults. Additionally, many teenagers use chewing tobacco or cigars, which can cause mouth cancer. Those most at risk are males in low-income families with parents who smoke. Male adolescents may smoke to be rebellious, but females often smoke to lose weight. Other factors include the desire to be part of a group, lack of supervision, and accessibility of tobacco. *Intervention* includes identifying those smoking, providing information about the dangers of smoking beginning with children at about 9 years old, and providing programs to help teenagers quit smoking.

Drug Use

Drug use continues to be a serious problem for children and teenagers, with some starting as young as 9 or 10, using a wide variety of drugs, including marijuana, crack, prescription drugs, cocaine, inhalants (such as glue and lighter fluid), hallucinogens, and steroids. Risk factors include aggressive behavior, poor social skills, and poor academic progress coupled with lack of parental supervision, poverty, and availability of drugs. Small children are often reacting to circumstances within the family while teenagers are responding to peer pressure from outside the family. Studies have shown that early *intervention* to teach children better self-control and coping skills is often more effective than trying to change behavior patterns that are established, so family-based programs often show positive results. Teenagers may need help with basic academic skills and social skills to improve communication. Methods of resisting drugs must be provided and reinforced. Drug recovery programs can be helpful but are often too expensive or not available for those who need them.

Alcohol Use

Alcohol is a significant problem in adolescence and even in younger children. It is the most-commonly abused substance. Studies have shown that about 32% of young people drink and 20% are binge drinkers. While alcohol can impair development of almost all body systems in a growing child, it is of particular concern for the effects on the neurological system and liver. Additionally, because it interferes with impulse control, adolescents who drink are often involved in violence, abuse, and at-risk sexual behavior. Drinking should be suspected if a child has memory problems, changes in behavior, poor academic progress, emotional lability, and physical changes, such as slurring of speech, general lethargy, or lack of coordination. *Intervention* includes teaching children from about age 9 about the dangers of drinking, identifying those who are drinking, identifying underlying problems, and providing programs to help teenagers stop drinking, such as counselling or Alcoholics Anonymous.

High-Risk Sexual Behavior

High-risk sexual behavior in teenagers is often coupled with other health-risk behaviors, such as drinking and drug use, and teenagers are having sex at younger ages. About 47% of high school seniors have had sex, with many beginning as young as 10-12 years. Risk factors include poverty, single-family homes, lack of supervision, and siblings or peers who are sexually active. Those who have sex before age 15 are especially vulnerable, often having multiple partners and unprotected sex, leading to sexually transmitted diseases (STDs) and pregnancy. They are emotionally vulnerable and often can't deal effectively with relationships. *Intervention* should begin early with age-appropriate honest sex education. Abstinence education, while the ideal, has not been successful in changing the sexual behavior of teenagers, with studies showing that many of those signing pledges to remain virgins are already sexually active. Teenagers who are sexually active should be advised regarding the use of condoms, birth control, and protection from STDs in a non-judgmental manner.

Prevention of STDs

The **CDC** has developed 5 strategies to **prevent** and **control** the spread of **STDs**:

- **Educate** those at risk about how to make changes in sexual practices to prevent infection.
- **Identify** symptomatic and asymptomatic infected persons who might not seek diagnosis or treatment.
- **Diagnose** and treat those who are infected.
- **Prevent infection** of sex partners through evaluation, treatment, and counseling.
- Provide pre-exposure **vaccination** for those at risk.

Practitioners are advised of patients' **sexual histories** and to assess risk. The 5-P approach to questioning is advocated. Practitioners should ask about:

- **Partners**: Gender and number.
- **Pregnancy** prevention: Birth control.
- **Protection**: Methods used.

- **Practices**: Type of sexual practices (oral, anal, vaginal) and use of condoms.
- **Past history of STDs**: High-risk behavior (promiscuity, prostitution) and disease risk (human immunodeficiency virus [HIV]/ hepatitis).

The **CDC** recommends a number of specific preventive methods as part of the clinical guidelines for **prevention of sexually transmitted diseases:**

- **Abstinence**/reduction in number of sex partners.
- Pre-exposure **vaccination**: All those evaluated for STDs should receive hepatitis B vaccination, and men who have sex with men (MSM) and illicit drug users should receive hepatitis A vaccination.
- **Male latex (or polyurethane) condoms** should be used for all sexual encounters with only water-based lubricants used with latex.
- **Female condoms** may be used if male condom cannot be used properly.
- Condoms and diaphragms should not be used with spermicides containing **nonoxynol-9 (N-9)**, and N-9 should not be used as a lubricant for anal sex.
- **Non-barrier contraceptive measures** provide no protection from STDs and must not be relied on to prevent disease.

Effects of Alternative Life-Style Choices on Health Risks

As young people become sexually active, most are attracted to members of the opposite sex, but others face **alternative lifestyle** choices:

- Gay and lesbian (homosexual) teenagers are attracted to members of their own sex while bisexual teenagers are attracted to both sexes. Between 1-10% of teenagers identify themselves as homosexual, often feeling different from a very young age. These adolescents are at increased risk of violence, sexual abuse, depression, and harassment. They may not be accepted by their families or friends and sometimes become homeless. They are at risk for STDs and HIV and suffer from high rates of suicide.
- Some children are transgender, sometimes identifying from preschool age with the opposite sex and choosing to live in that role. They often suffer much prejudice because there is little understanding of transgender issues.

Intervention includes providing support and acceptance as well as practical assistance for housing, safe-sex instruction, counseling, and support groups.

Common Injuries to Infants and Children and Prevention Strategies

Injuries are a concern for infants and small children, who are particularly vulnerable to injury because they are not able to protect themselves, but older children often engage in activities that pose serious dangers:

- *Neck/head injuries,* especially in neonates, are caused by lack of support. Parents should be advised to support the neck or young infant and to avoid shaking or throwing infant. Older children should be supervised when holding infants.
- *Aspiration* can occur because of the strong sucking reflex in small infants and later when the child picks up and puts small objects in the mouth. Guidelines for feeding and home and toy safety should be provided to all parents.

- *Hypothermia* most often occurs because people fail to provide adequate clothing or covering for children in cold climates or when children wander outside in cold weather. Outside doors should be locked so that children cannot open then or preventive knob covers installed.
- *Hyperthermia* may occur if children are outside for long periods or left in cars. Parent should be advised that children have poor temperature control and cannot handle extremes of temperature well and should NEVER be left alone in a motor vehicle, even on cool days.
- *Poisoning* frequently occurs because medications or toxic substances are left within reach of small children, whose taste senses have not fully developed so that they drink foul-tasting liquids. All medications should be out of reach and cleaning and other chemicals placed in upper cabinets and/or secured cabinets.
- *Falls and subsequent injuries* occur when walkers tip over and when children begins to walk and trip over things, falls down stairs, or falls into sharp objects or corners of furniture. Children should be supervised at all times, doors to stairways secured, and sharp corners padded. Children should not use walkers. Children may also pull things on themselves, causing injury, so the environment should be childproofed.
- *Drowning* usually occurs when children are left unsupervised in a bath, left in a bath with young siblings, or fall into swimming pools or bodies of water. Parents should never assume that telling a child "no, no" or warning them against going near a swimming pool repeatedly is going to protect a small child from danger as children lack impulse control and internalization of cause-effect.
- *Trauma* from motor vehicle accidents, either as a passenger, drivers, or pedestrians, is common for all ages. Proper safety seats and safety restraints of the children provide the best preventive methods for passengers. Small children should be taught about safely crossing the street and to avoid running in traffic, but they should never be trusted to cross the street without supervision until school age. They should not play in an unfenced yard with access to the street without close supervision as children may run in front of traffic.
- *Sports injuries* become more common as children participate in team sports or individual activities with higher risks, such as skiing and skateboarding. Wheeled shoes also cause many injuries. Children should have supervised strength training and play in age-appropriate supervised sports. Football is the most dangerous team sport and is not appropriate for young children. Children should wear proper equipment, including padding and helmets, while playing sports. Bicyclists have increased risk because of traffic and should always wear proper helmets.
- *Drug overdoses* are most commonly from the use of illicit drugs during adolescence. Complex socio-behavioral forces are involved, and preventive measure must start early to identify those at risk. Sometimes younger children are also involved in huffing, inhaling of substances such as glue and lighter fluid, which can lead to death. Dangerous fads often occur among teenagers, and parents and the APRN should remain aware of problems in the community so that they can address the matter with the children.

Age-Appropriate Counseling

Substance Use

Alcohol Use in Children/Adolescents

Alcohol is a significant problem in adolescence and even in younger children. It is the most commonly abused substance. Studies have shown that about 32% of young people drink and 20% are binge drinkers. While alcohol can impair development of almost all body systems in a growing child, it is of particular concern for the effects on the **neurological system and liver**. Additionally, because it interferes with impulse control, adolescents who drink are often involved in violence, abuse, and at-risk sexual behavior. Drinking should be expected if a child has memory problems, changes in behavior, poor academic progress, emotional lability, and physical changes, such as slurring of speech, general lethargy, or lack of coordination. *Intervention* includes teaching children from about age 9 about the dangers of drinking, identifying those who are drinking, identifying underlying problems, and providing programs to help teenagers stop drinking, such as counseling or Alcoholics Anonymous.

Drug Use in Children and Adolescents

Drug use continues to be a serious problem for children and teenagers, with some starting as young as 9 or 10, using a wide variety of drugs, including marijuana, crack, prescription drugs, cocaine, inhalants (such as glue and lighter fluid), hallucinogens, and steroids. Risk factors include aggressive behavior, poor social skills, and poor academic progress coupled with lack of parental supervision, poverty, and availability of drugs. Small children are often reacting to circumstances **within the family** while teenagers are responding to peer pressure from **outside the family**. Studies have shown that **early intervention** to teach children better self-control and coping skills is often more effective than trying to change behavior patterns that are established, so family-based programs often show positive results. Teenagers may need help with basic academic skills and social skills to improve communication. Methods of resisting drugs must be provided and reinforced. Drug recovery programs can be helpful but are often too expensive or not available for those who need them.

Indicators of Substance Abuse

Many people with substance abuse (alcohol or drugs) are reluctant to disclose this information, but there are a number of indicators that are suggestive of **substance abuse:**

Physical signs	Other signs
Needle tracks on arms or legs.	Odor of alcohol/marijuana on clothing or breath.
Burns on fingers or lips.	Labile emotions, including mood swings, agitation, and anger.
Pupils abnormally dilated or constricted, eyes watery.	Inappropriate, impulsive, and/or risky behavior.
Slurring of speech, slow speech.	Lying.
Lack of coordination, instability of gait.	Missing appointments.
Tremors.	Difficulty concentrating/short term memory loss, disoriented/confused.
Sniffing repeatedly, nasal irritation.	Blackouts.
Persistent cough.	Insomnia or excessive sleeping.
Weight loss.	Lack of personal hygiene.
Dysrhythmias.	
Pallor, puffiness of face.	

Ethanol Overdose

Ethanol is the form of alcohol found in alcoholic beverages, flavorings, and some medications. Ethanol overdose is responsible for about 8000 deaths of children and teenagers each year. Ingestion in small children is often accidental, but teenagers frequently use ethanol as a drug of choice and binge drinking can lead to serious morbidity or death. Ethanol has direct effects of the central nervous system, myocardium, thyroid, and hepatic tissue. Ethanol is absorbed through the mucosa of the mouth, stomach, and intestines, with concentrations peaking about 30-60 minutes after ingestion. About 90% of ethanol is metabolized in the liver and the rest excreted through the pulmonary and renal systems. In children, the liver clears ethanol more rapidly than in adults, at about 30 mg/dL/hr or about 0.5 ounce/hr. combining drugs with alcohol potentiates the effects. Some children and teenagers may develop toxicity at lower levels of ethanol ingestion than other.

Symptoms and Treatment

Ethanol overdose affects young children differently than teenagers or adults. Additionally, young children often ingest alcohol in products such as perfumes and cleaning solutions, which are often more toxic than beer or alcoholic beverages.

- Infants and young children:
  - Seizures and coma. Respiratory depression and hypoxia. Hypoglycemia (especially infants and toddlers). Hypothermia.
- Teenagers:
  - Altered mental status. Hypotension. Bradycardia with arrhythmias. Respiratory depression and hypoxia.
  - Cold, clammy skin or flushed skin (from vasodilation). Acute pancreatitis with abdominal pain. Lack of consciousness.
  - Circulatory collapse leading to death.

Treatment includes:

- Careful monitoring of arterial blood gases and oxygen saturation.
- Ensure patent airway with intubation and ventilation if necessary.
- Intravenous fluids.
- Dextrose to correct hypoglycemia if indicated.
- Maintain body temperature (warming blanket).
- Dialysis may be necessary in severe cases.

Management of Bereavement

Bereavement occurs after the death of family, friend, or someone to whom a person identifies closely. It is a time of mourning and is part of the natural grieving process, but some people are not able to move past the grieving discuss process and may suffer signs related to depression, such as poor appetite, insomnia, and other symptoms, such as chest pain, that may mimic physical illnesses. Some may enter a stage of denial or anger that interferes with their daily activities and work. People suffering bereavement may present with vague and varied complaints. A careful history is important. *Treatment* varies according to the needs of the individual. In some cases, selective serotonin reuptake inhibitors (SSRIs, such as Prozac® [fluoxetine]) may provide temporary relief, but the patient should be referred for psychological counselling, bereavement services, or psychiatric care, depending upon the severity of symptoms.

Assessment and Diagnosis

Comprehensive Health Assessment

Assessing History for Genetic or Familial Risks

Assessing family history for **genetic or familial risks** is an important part of disease prevention because, in some cases, early identification and intervention may reduce future health risks. Creating a genogram with the family is helpful. A thorough history should be broad and include assessment of the following:

- Early onset disorders, such as cardiovascular disease, hypertension, or Alzheimer's disease.
- Progressive neurological or neuromuscular diseases.
- Diabetes Mellitus.
- Mental illness, such as depression, bipolar disorder, and schizophrenia.
- Intellectual disability, including Trisomy 21 (Down syndrome).
- Any unusual disabilities or abnormalities, such as birth defects.

Once risk factors are determined, then the question of screening tests arises. If there is a possibility that the child is a carrier, then screening is usually deferred until the child can give informed consent. Screening is done with parental permission when it is in the best interests of the child, allowing for appropriate care and intervention.

Relationship of Ethnicity to Increased Risk of Genetic Disorders

Some ethnic groups have increased risk for **genetic disorders** with high carrier rates, ranging from 1:6-1:40. The nurse practitioner should be aware of these risks and observant for symptoms in the child. A careful maternal and paternal family history may provide information about occurrence of the disease in other family members. Some disorders are covered in routine neonatal screening, but others are not. In some cases, it may be appropriate to recommend testing to ensure that early diagnosis is made so that treatment can be initiated. The following groups are at increased risk for specific genetic disorders:

- Ashkenazi Jews: Canavan disease, Tay Sachs disease, cystic fibrosis, and familial dysautonomia.
- African Americans: Sickle cell disease (carrier rate 1:6-12), other hemoglobinopathy.
- European Caucasians: cystic fibrosis.
- Mediterranean: Beta thalassemia.
- South Asian: Beta Thalassemia.
- Southeast Asian: Alpha and Beta Thalassemia.

Review of Systems: Respiratory

Functions of the Respiratory Tract

The basic functions of the respiratory tract include:

- *Gas exchange:* Oxygen is transported into the cells where it is exchanged in the capillaries for carbon dioxide.
- *Respiration:* The process by which gas exchange between outside air and the blood and then between the blood and cells takes place is the respiration cycle.
- *Ventilation:* Physical factors that govern air flow include:
  - Air pressure variances: air flows from areas of greater pressure to areas of lower pressure.
  - Airway resistance: the relationship between the size of the airway and the amount of airflow.
  - Compliance: the volume-pressure relationship in the lungs and thorax that allows the lungs and thorax to stretch and distend (comply) under pressure. Compliance increases with loss of elasticity and distended thorax (emphysema) and decreases with increased "stiffness" or resistance in the lungs and thorax (pneumothorax, hemothorax, ARDS, fibrosis, and atelectasis).

Anatomy and Function of the Upper Respiratory Tract

Nose and Paranasal Sinuses

The **upper respiratory tract** comprises the nose and nasal passages, the sinuses, the pharynx, tonsils, adenoids, larynx, and trachea.

- *The nose* serves as the passageway for air to pass into and out of the lungs. The nares open on the outside. Internally, the septum divides the passage into a right and left nasal cavity, which are further divided by the turbinate bones projecting laterally from the walls into 3 passages on each side. The turbinate bones (conchae) deflect the air to the superior aspect of the nasal cavities, increasing air contact with mucous membranes to help filter dust and organisms. The nasal cavities are lined with mucosa, coated with mucus and cilia to move the debris to the nasopharynx. The mucous membrane also warms and moistens the air. The olfactory receptors are located in the mucosa as well.
- *The paranasal sinuses* are 4 mucosa-lined bony cavities that serve as resonating chambers for production of speech: frontal, ethmoidal, sphenoidal, and maxillary.

Pharynx, Tonsils, Adenoids, Larynx, and Trachea

The **upper respiratory tract**:

- *The pharynx* is the throat and is divided into 3 sections: the nasopharynx is posterior to the nose and superior to the soft palate and contains the adenoids (pharyngeal tonsils); the oropharynx is posterior to the tongue and houses the palatine (faucial) tonsils. The laryngopharynx extends posteriorly from the hyoid bone to the cricoid cartilage with the epiglottis separating the pharynx from the larynx. The pharynx serves as the passageway for both the respiratory and gastrointestinal tracts.

- *The larynx* is a cartilaginous structure that aids vocalization and facilitates coughing. It contains the epiglottis, the glottis, the thyroid cartilage, the cricoid cartilage, and the arytenoid cartilage as well as the vocal cords.
- *The trachea* carries air from the larynx to the bronchi and protected by anterior C-shaped cartilaginous rings that provide structure.

Anatomy and Function of the Lower Respiratory Tract

Lungs

The lungs consist of a pair of elastic organs inside the thoracic cage, with the diaphragmatic muscle at the base, creating an airtight space with distensible walls. During ventilation, the walls distend and the pressure inside lowers so air passes into the lungs (inspiration). The air causes an increase in pressure, and the thoracic cage contracts and the lungs force air out (expiration). The thorax and lungs are lined with a serous membrane containing pleural fluid to prevent friction during ventilation. The mediastinum is between the lungs, extending from the sternum to the vertebrae. Each lung is divided into lobes: 2 on the left and 3 on the right, and each lobe is further divided into 2-5 segments. The bronchi that carry oxygen to the lungs are divided into lobar, segmental, subsegmental, and bronchioles (which have no cartilage). The bronchioles then divide into terminal bronchioles (with no mucus or cilia), to respiratory bronchioles to alveolar ducts, alveolar sacs, and alveoli, where gas exchange occurs.

Clinical Indications of Acute Respiratory Infections

Fever, Lymph Nodes, and Meningeal Irritation
Children with **acute respiratory infections** may manifest a wide range of symptoms:

- *Fever* is usually absent in neonates but is highest in those from 6 months to 3 years of age, and may reach 103-105 °F. Sudden temperature rises to 104° may result in seizures in children <3-4 years of age. Fever may result in some children being listless and others hyperactive.
- *Cervical lymph nodes* may be tender and enlarged.
- *Meningeal irritation* occurs in some children without meningitis in the presence of an abrupt increase in fever and may manifest with headaches, nuchal rigidity and pain, as well as positive Kernig and Brudzinski signs.
  - Positive Kernig's sign: Flex each hip and then try to straighten the knee while the hip is flexed. Spasm of the hamstrings makes this painful and difficult.
  - Brudzinski sign: With child lying supine, flex the neck by pulling head toward chest. The neck stiffness causes the hips and knees to pull up into a flexed position.

Nasal and Respiratory Symptoms
Nasal and respiratory symptoms are indicative of **acute respiratory infection**:

- *Nasal symptoms* may include swelling of nasal passages, causing obstruction that can interfere with feeding in small infants. Exudate may be thin and watery or thick and purulent, depending upon the type of infection. Irritation about the nares and upper lip related to exudate is common in infants and small children.
- *Sore throat* is usually a complaint of older children. Small infants and children may have an inflamed throat but appear to suffer less discomfort.
- *Cough* is a common symptom that may occur only during the acute phase of the respiratory infection or may persist for months after initial infection.

69

- *Change in respiratory sounds* may include wheezing and hoarseness in addition to cough. On auscultation, abnormal sounds may occur, such as hyperresonance, fine to coarse rales, wheezing, or absence of breath sounds in areas of the lungs.

Gastrointestinal Disorders

Children with **respiratory infections** may initially manifest with gastrointestinal symptoms:

- *Poor appetite* or poor feeding is often the initial symptom and may persist throughout the febrile and convalescent period. This is a common symptom of acute infection in children.
- *Nausea and vomiting* may occur before other symptoms by several hours and usually subsides fairly quickly although it may persist with some children. It is most common in small children.
- *Diarrhea* is common with respiratory infections, especially those of viral origin. In most children it is mild and short lasting, but in others it may be severe and increase dehydration.
- *Abdominal pain* may be related to muscle spasms from vomiting or lymphadenitis of mesentery, especially if the child is very tense. The type of pain may be similar to or indistinguishable from pain associated with appendicitis.

Lower Respiratory Tract Infections

Bronchitis

Bronchitis is inflammation of the trachea and bronchi (tracheobronchial tree) and is common in children to age 4. It often occurs as a progression of an upper respiratory infection, so upper respiratory symptoms may also be evident. Bronchitis is usually caused by viruses, but can also be caused by bacteria and fungi. *Mycoplasma pneumoniae* is often implicated in children over age 6. Viral bronchitis is usually essentially a mild, self-limiting disorder characterized by a dry, hacking cough that usually worsens at night and is productive within 2-3 days of onset. It clears within 5-10 days. Bronchitis of longer duration may not be viral and should be evaluated with sputum cultures.

Treatment is usually symptomatic and includes:

- Analgesics.
- Antipyretics.
- Cough suppressants and cough expectorants. Cough suppressants should be used sparingly at night to allow rest, but may thicken secretions and prolong symptoms.
- Antibiotics are NOT indicated for viral bronchitis.

Bronchiolitis

Bronchiolitis is inflammation of the bronchiolar level and is usually caused by the **respiratory syncytial virus (RSV)** although adenoviruses, parainfluenza and *M. pneumoniae* have also been implicated. It is most common in very small children between the ages of 2 months and 2 years and rarely occurs after that age. Most children who require hospitalization are infants under 6 months of age. The infection is usually seasonal and is usually mild although it can result in severe respiratory complications so children should be observed carefully. Symptoms include dyspnea, a paroxysmal cough that is non-productive, tachypnea and wheezing. The infection is usually self-limiting and runs its course in 8-15 days but is highly contagious.

Treatment is usually symptomatic and includes:

- *Antipyretics*, such as acetaminophen.
- *Oxygen therapy* with intubation and mechanical ventilation may be required in the presence of severe disease and respiratory compromise.
- *Ribavirin* aerosol is used for severe disease.

Pneumonia

Pneumonia is inflammation of the lung parenchyma, filling the alveoli with exudate. It is common throughout childhood and adulthood but more frequent in infants and young children. Pneumonia may be a primary disease or may occur secondary to another infection or disease, such as lung cancer. It may be caused by bacteria, viruses, parasites, or fungi. It may also be caused by chemical damage. Pneumonia is characterized by location:

- *Lobar* involves one or more lobes of the lungs. If lobes in both lungs are affected, it is referred to as "bilateral" or "double" pneumonia.
- *Bronchial/lobular* involves the terminal bronchioles and exudate can involve the adjacent lobules. Usually the pneumonia occurs in scattered patches throughout the lungs.
- *Interstitial* involves primarily the interstitium and alveoli where white blood cells and plasma fill the alveoli, generating inflammation and creating fibrotic tissue as the alveoli are destroyed.

Viral Pneumonia

Viral pneumonia is more common in adults than children although the respiratory syncytial virus (RSV), which causes upper respiratory infections and bronchiolitis can progress to pneumonia and is most commonly found in children ≤5. A number of other viruses, such as adenoviruses, parainfluenza, cytomegalovirus, and coronavirus may be implicated. The viruses invade the cells that line the airways and alveoli, causing death of the cells. *Symptoms* related to viral pneumonia are similar to those of bacterial pneumonia although the onset is often slow with pneumonia preceded by a respiratory infection that progressively worsens, with increasing cough, fever, dyspnea, cyanosis, and respiratory distress. There are few effective treatments for viral pneumonia, and one danger is that a viral pneumonia increases susceptibility to bacterial infection of the lungs. **Treatment** may include:

Rest and adequate fluids and nutrition.
- *Antipyretics*, such as acetaminophen.
- *Oxygen therapy* with intubation and mechanical ventilation may be required in the presence of severe disease and respiratory compromise.
- *Ribavirin* aerosol is used for severe RSV disease and pneumonia.

Community-Acquired Pneumonia

Hemophilus Influenzae

Hemophilus influenzae frequently colonizes the upper respiratory tracts in children <5 and can lead to pneumonia. However, in 1990, the conjugated polysaccharide *H. influenza* type b vaccine was introduced, and this has greatly decreased the incidence of pneumonia in small children. Non-type B and non-typeable cases of *H. influenzae* pneumonia do occur. This pneumonia is similar in symptoms to other bacterial forms, but the onset if often slow and insidious, appearing 2-6 weeks after an upper respiratory tract infection. *Symptoms* include fever, chills, and productive cough. The disease may occur as lobar or bronchial pneumonia or with areas of consolidation where the alveoli have collapsed and the tissue hardened. Complications may include bacteremia, lung abscesses, pleural effusions, epiglottitis, and pericarditis. **Treatment** is symptomatic and may include:

- Antipyretics.
- Analgesics.
- Respiratory support.
- Antibiotics: Ampicillin, 3ʳᵈ generation cephalosporin, macrolides.

Streptococcus Pneumoniae

Streptococcus pneumoniae (a Gram-positive coccus) is part of the normal flora of the upper respiratory tract and is the most frequent cause of bacterial pneumonia, often secondary to an upper respiratory tract infection. The overall incidence has dropped since the heptavalent pneumococcal conjugate vaccine (PCV-7) was introduced in 2000, with the most significant effect on those under 2 years of age (78% drop in cases); however, a vaccinated infant that is febrile with toxic symptoms and a leukocyte count of ≥15,000 cells/mL is at risk for pneumonia. The bacteria induce an acute inflammatory response causing the alveoli and interstitium to fill with protein-rich fluid. The infection spreads quickly, often to multiple lobes, causing consolidation, pleural effusions, super infections, bacteremia (15-25%) and pericarditis may occur. *Symptoms* include an abrupt onset with high fever (≥105 °F), chills, diaphoresis, cyanosis, chest pain, tachypnea, tachycardia, altered consciousness, and cough productive of rusty or green-tinged mucus. **Treatment** may include:

- Antipyretics.
- Analgesics.
- Respiratory support.
- Antibiotics: penicillins or others.

Mycoplasma Pneumoniae

Mycoplasma pneumoniae is caused by pleomorphic (variously shaped) microorganisms that interfere with the function of the cilia and produce hydrogen peroxide, which disrupts cell functions. They also activate an inflammatory response. Only about 3% of those infected develop pneumonia, affecting primarily children and young adults between the ages of 4 and 20. Mycoplasma pneumoniae occurs seasonally in the fall in a regular 4-8-year cycle of epidemics. The onset is usually gradual, and children tend to be less obviously ill than with other types of pneumonia. Symptoms may include a paroxysmal cough, low-grade fever, myalgia, diarrhea, erythematous rash and pharyngitis. The pneumonia presents as interstitial infiltrates on x-ray. While complications, such as myocarditis, endocarditis, and aseptic meningitis and encephalitis may occur, most infections clear without sequelae. **Treatment** includes;

- *Antibiotic therapy:* Erythromycin, tetracycline, macrolide, or fluoroquinolone.
- *Symptomatic support:* Antidiarrheals, antipyretics, and analgesics.

Periodic Breathing

Periodic breathing may occur in both premature and full-term neonates.

With **symptoms** of periodic breathing, normal periods of respirations lasting 20 seconds or longer are followed by periods of apnea that may last up to 10 seconds, occurring 3 or more times in succession, followed by a period of hyperventilation. However, there is no concomitant cyanosis or significant bradycardia or decrease in oxygen saturation, which occurs with apnea of prematurity.

Periodic breathing does not occur until 2 days after birth. Periodic breathing occurs in 2-6% of the respirations of full-term infants but increases to up to 25% of respirations for premature infants. It occurs more frequently during active sleep than while the child is awake and may occur at high altitudes. **Treatment** is usually not necessary although oxygen or continuous positive airway pressure (CPAP) may be administered for infants exhibiting periodic breathing at high altitudes.

Review of Systems: EENT

Infectious Conjunctivitis

Infectious conjunctivitis (pink eye) is inflammation of the conjunctiva of the eye from bacteria or viruses. If it occurs <30 days of birth, it is referred to as *ophthalmia neonatorum* and is commonly acquired during delivery:

- Pathogenic agents include *Chlamydia trachomatis, Neisseria gonorrhea,* and herpesvirus.
- Antibiotic drops are applied to the newborns eyes to prevent conjunctivitis. Intravenous acyclovir is given to infants exposed to herpes virus.

Infectious conjunctivitis in older children is usually caused by *Staphylococci, Streptococci, Pneumococci* or viruses and is extremely contagious, so good hand hygiene is essential. It is difficult to differentiate between bacterial and viral infections without cultures. The child should be kept from school and other children for 24 hours after starting treatment or until **symptoms** subside:

* Red, swollen, itchy conjunctiva. * Eye pain. * Purulent discharge. * Scratchy feeling under eyelids. * Mild photophobia.

Treatment is usually antibiotic drops or ointment and cool compresses although many cases are caused by viruses and the condition often disappears without treatment in 3-5 days.

Strabismus

Strabismus occurs when the muscles of the eyes are not coordinated so that one eye deviates from the axis of the other. Strabismus may be congenital or acquired or associated with other disorders, such as albinism. Deviations include:

- *Phoria* is intermittent deviation but the child can focus eyes and maintain alignment for periods when looking at an object.
- *Tropia* is consistent or intermittent deviation in which the child is unable to maintain alignment of the eyes.
- Both phorias and tropias may be *hyper* (up), *hypo* (down), *exo* (out), *eso* (in toward nose), or *cyclo* (rotational).

Esotropia is both eyes turning inwards (cross eyes) and *exotropia* is both eyes turning outward (wall eyes). Children often compensate by closing one eye or moving head. They may have headache or dizziness. **Treatment** <24 months reduces *amblyopia* (reduced vision):

- Occlusion therapy: patching or eye drops to blur vision in one eye.
- Eye exercises.
- Corrective lenses and/or prisms.
- Surgical repair of rectus muscle.

Retinopathy of Prematurity

Retinopathy of prematurity (ROP) occurs when small capillaries to the retina constrict, causing necrosis. ROP is associated with infants born ≤28 week and weighing <1600 g (3lb. 8 oz), especially those receiving oxygen therapy. It is also linked to respiratory distress, hypoxia, hypercarbia, acidosis, shock, blood transfusions, and systemic infection. In many cases, revascularization will occur, but ROP may result in myopia, retinal detachment, and blindness. Infants at risk for ROP should have regular evaluations for visual impairment:

- Infants may be unable to follow objects or lights with eyes, fail to make eye contact or imitate facial expressions. They may have a vacant stare.
- Toddlers and young children may thrust head forward, hold objects close to eyes, squint or blink frequently, rub or cover eyes, and bump into objects.

Treatment includes:

- Corrective lenses.
- Cryosurgery or laser surgery to stop disease progression.
- Scleral buckle procedure or vitrectomy may be indicated for retinal detachment.

Glaucoma

Glaucoma is an increase in intraocular pressure caused by abnormal circulation of fluid in the eyes: the ciliary body of the eyes produces aqueous fluid that flows between the iris and lens to the anterior chamber where it collects and increases pressure, which can result in blindness. Glaucoma may affect one eye or both. There are 2 types:

- *Congenital glaucoma* occurs < 3 years and includes an abnormality of structures that drain aqueous humor. Treatment is often unsuccessful. Symptoms include:
  o Photophobia
  o Tearing
  o Clouding of cornea
  o Eyelid spasms and enlargement of eyes
- *Secondary/juvenile glaucoma* occurs >3 years and is caused by obstruction related to trauma, infection, tumors, or steroid use. Secondary glaucoma symptoms may be less specific: Bumping into objects because of loss of visual field and seeing halos about objects.

Treatment includes:

- Eye drops used for adults are relatively ineffective for children.
- Surgical reduction of pressure is treatment of choice, and the child may require multiple procedures.

Cataracts

Cataracts, partial or complete opacity of the lens of one or both eyes preventing refraction of light onto the retina, can be either congenital or acquired and is associated with prenatal infections, (such as rubella and CMV), hypocalcemia, or drug exposure. It can be related to trauma, systemic corticosteroids, genetic defects (albinism, Down syndrome) and prematurity. Clouding of the lens is not always obvious to the naked eye, so careful visual evaluations should be done for those children at risk. **Treatment** depends upon the extent of the cataracts and whether they are unilateral or

74

bilateral. Early diagnosis is important because surgical repair ≤2 months is the most successful with visual acuity in 55% at 20/40. The opaque lens is removed and the child uses corrective lenses or a lens is implanted. Antibiotic or steroid drops may be used after surgery.

Nystagmus and Blepharoptosis

Nystagmus is involuntary rhythmic movements of one or both eyes, with horizontal, vertical, or circular movements, sometimes accompanied by rhythmic movements of the head. Nystagmus is common in neonates and should resolve in a few weeks but may indicate pathology if it persists. It is often associated with albinism, CNS abnormalities, or diseases of the ear or retina, and sudden onset is cause for concern. There is no specific treatment other than to identify and treat underlying causes.

Blepharoptosis is drooping of one or both upper eyelids and may be congenital (autosomal dominant), with defective development of the levator muscles or cranial nerve III, or acquired as the result of trauma or infection. If vision is affected, surgical repair is done early to avoid amblyopia. If vision is unaffected, surgical repair is deferred until the child is 3 or older.

Normal Hearing Developmental Characteristics Used to Assess Hearing Deficits in Infants and Toddlers

Hearing deficits may be identified very early if developmental characteristics are carefully observed in infants and children. **Normal hearing** responses include:

- ≤3 months: Positive Moro (startle) reflex to sound. Noise disturbs sleep, and reacts to sounds by opening eyes or blinking.
- 3-6 months: Comforts at sound of parent's voice and tries to emulate sounds. Looks in the direction of sound.
- 6-12 months: Begins to vocalize more with cooing and gurgling with different inflections. Responds to name and simple words and looks in the direction of sound.
- 12-18 months: Begins first words about 12-15 months and imitates sounds, follows vocal directions, and points to familiar items when asked.
- 18-24 months: More verbal with about half of vocabulary understandable and knows about 20-50 words. Points to body parts of familiar objects with asked.

Hearing Loss

Identifying **hearing loss** early can facilitate treatment and prevent further deterioration, but most children are not diagnosed until 14-24 months even if hearing loss is profound and diagnosis is delayed ≤48 months for less severe hearing loss:

- Mild hearing loss: pure-tone loss of ≥40 decibels at 500, 1000, and 2000 Hz in the better ear.
- Moderate: 40-60 decibel loss.
- Severe: 60-80 decibel loss.
- Profound: ≥80 decibel.

There are 3 types of hearing loss:

- *Sensorineural hearing loss (SNHL):* Damage occurs to the cochlear structure or nerve fibers. Hearing loss is permanent and associated with genetic disorders, birth injury, toxic drugs, head trauma, neoplasms, and viruses. A sub-form is noise-induced hearing loss (NIHL), which is preventable, but also permanent.

- *Conductive hearing loss (CHL):* Transmission of sound is blocked by infection, foreign object, debris, impacted cerumen, and neoplasms. This type of hearing loss is usually reversible with medication or surgery.
- *Mixed hearing loss (MHL):* Both conductive and sensorial loss.

Otitis Externa

Otitis externa (OE) is infection of the external ear canal, either bacterial or mycotic. Common pathogens include bacteria, *Pseudomonas aeruginosa, Staphylococcus aureus,* and fungi, *Aspergillus* and *Candida.* OE is often caused by chlorine in swimming pools killing normal flora and allowing other bacteria to multiply. Fungal infections may be associated with immune disorders, diabetes, and steroid use. **Symptoms** include:

- Pain, swelling, and exudate.
- Itching (pronounced with fungal infections).
- Red pustular lesions.
- Black spots over tympanic membrane (fungus).

Treatment includes:

- Irrigate ear with Burrows solution or saline to clean and remove debris, foreign objects.
- Bacteria: Antibiotic ear drops, such as ciprofloxacin and ofloxacin. If impetigo, flush with hydrogen peroxide 1:1 solution and apply Bactroban® twice daily for 5-7 days. Lance pointed furuncles.
- Fungus: Solution of 5% boric acid in ethanol; Clotrimazole-miconazole solution with/without steroid for 5-7 days.
- Analgesics as needed.

Otitis Media

Otitis media, inflammation of the middle ear, usually follows upper respiratory infections or allergic rhinitis. The Eustachian tube swells and prevents the passage of air. Fluid from the mucous membranes pools in the middle ear, causing infection. Common pathogens include *Streptococcus pneumoniae, Haemophilus influenzae,* and *Moraxella catarrhalis.* Some genetic conditions, such as trisomy 21 and cleft palate may include abnormalities of the Eustachian tube, increasing risk. There are 4 forms:

- Acute: 1-3 weeks with swelling, redness, and possible rupture of the tympanic membrane, fever, pain (ear pulling), and hearing loss.
- Recurrent: 3 episodes in 6 months or 4-6 in 12.
- Bullous: Acute infection with ear popping pressure in middle ear, pain, hearing loss, and bullae between layers of tympanic membrane, causing bulging.
- Chronic: Persists ≥3 months with thick retracted tympanic membrane, hearing loss, and drainage.

Treatment includes:

- 75-90% resolve spontaneously so antibiotics are withheld for 2-3 days.
- Amoxicillin for 7-10 days.
- Tympanostomy and pressure-equalizing tubes (PET) for severe chronic or recurrent infections.

Cochlear Implants

While there has been controversy in the deaf community about cochlear implants, by 2005, 22,000 children in the United States had received them. A **cochlea implant** is an electronic device that provides sound, although not normal hearing, to those who have profound deafness. The person with the implant can often learn to understand speech and environmental sounds. Some use the sounds with lip-reading, but about half are able to understand speech by sound only, depending upon the degree of damage to the auditory nerve. A microphone by the ear picks up sounds that travels to an external speech processor and transmitter, which sends sounds to an implanted receiver where the sound is converted into electrical impulses sent to an internal electrode array implanted in the cochlea. The electrodes send the impulses to the auditory nerve, creating a perception of sound. Some children now receive bilateral cochlear implants. Studies show infants receiving the implant ≤age 2 acquire normal speech more rapidly than those implanted later.

Recurrent Epistaxis

Recurrent epistaxis is common in young children (over 2), especially boys, and is often related to nose picking, dry climate, or central heating in the winter. Kiesselbach's plexus in the anterior nares has plentiful vessels and bleeds easily. Bleeding in the posterior nares is more dangerous and can result in considerable blood loss. Bleeding from the anterior nares is usually confined to one nostril, but from the posterior nares, blood may flow through both nostrils or backward into the throat and the child may be observed swallowing. Teenagers abusing cocaine may suffer nosebleeds because of damage to the mucosa. Hematocrit and hemoglobin should be done to determine if blood loss is significant. Bleeding should stop within 20 minutes. **Treatment**:

- Child in upright position, leaning forward so blood doesn't flow down throat.
- Apply firm pressure below the nares or by pinching the nostrils firmly for 10 minutes.
- Severe bleeding may require packing and/or topical vasoconstrictors.
- Humidifiers may decrease irritation.

Review of Systems: Gastrointestinal

Acute Gastrointestinal Bleeding

Gastrointestinal bleeding is unusual in children, but the age of the child and symptoms can indicate the area that is bleeding:

- *Neonates:* Apparent bleeding may occur from the infant swallowing maternal blood during delivery or from allergy to milk protein, but actual bleeding may result from mucosal erosion from increased gastric acid or from maternal medications (aspirin, Phenobarbital) that cause problems with coagulation, or medications to the infant, such as indomethacin and dexamethasone. Bleeding indicates necrotizing enterocolitis, Hirschsprung's disease, volvulus, or coagulopathies.
- *Older infants*: Intussusception and mucosal lesions cause most bleeding.
- *Children/adolescents:* Wide range of disorders may cause bleeding, including ulcers, inflammatory bowel disease, infectious diarrhea. Stress ulcers may relate to system disease.

Symptoms include:

- Vomiting blood.
- Bloody or tarry stools.

- Abdominal distention.
- Hypotension with tachycardia.

Treatment includes:

- Fluid replacement with transfusions is necessary.
- Identification and treatment of underlying problem.
- Endoscopy or push enteroscopy for upper GI bleeding.
- Colonoscopy for lower GI bleeding.

Hypertrophic Pyloric Stenosis

Hypertrophic pyloric stenosis (PS) is obstruction of the pyloric sphincter between the gastric pylorus and small intestine, caused by hypertrophy and hyperplasia of the circular muscle of the pylorus so the enlarged tissue obstructs the sphincter. PS is more common in boys than girls and has a genetic predisposition. Onset of **symptoms** is usually >3 weeks:

- Projectile vomiting (1-4 feet) usually shortly after eating but may be delayed for a few hours. Emesis may be blood-tinged but non-bilious.
- Child is hungry and eats readily, but shows weight loss and sings of dehydration.
- Upper abdominal distention with palpable mass in epigastrium (to right of umbilicus).
- Visible left to right peristaltic waves.

Diagnosis is based on ultrasound. Decreased sodium and potassium levels may not be evident with dehydration.

Treatment includes:

- Intravenous fluids to restore hydration and electrolyte balance.
- Surgical pyloromyotomy: longitudinal incisions through the circular muscle fibers down to the submucosa to release the restriction and allow the muscle to expand.

Bowel Obstruction and Infarction

Bowel obstruction occurs when there is a mechanical obstruction of the passage of intestinal contents because of constriction of the lumen, occlusion of the lumen, or lack of muscular contractions (paralytic ileus). Obstruction may be caused by congenital or acquired abnormalities/disorders. **Symptoms** include:

- Abdominal pain and distention.
- Abdominal rigidity.
- Vomiting and dehydration.
- Diminished or no bowel sounds.
- Severe constipation (obstipation).
- Respiratory distress from diaphragm pushing against pleural cavity.
- Shock as plasma volume diminishes and electrolytes enter intestines from bloodstream.
- Sepsis as bacteria proliferates in bowel and invade bloodstream.

Bowel infarction is ischemia of the intestines related to severely restricted blood supply. It can be the result of a number of different conditions, such as volvulus and malrotation defects, and may follow untreated bowel obstruction. Children present with acute abdomen and shock, and mortality rates are very high even with resection of infarcted bowel.

78

Malrotation/Volvulus

Malrotation is a congenital defect in which the intestines are attached to the back of the abdominal wall by one single attachment rather than a broad band of attachments across the abdomen, essentially suspending the bowels so that they can easily twist, resulting in a **volvulus** (twisted bowel), cutting off blood supply. It may untwist but can lead to bowel infarction. Some children with malrotation have no symptoms, but most develop **symptoms** by 1 year:

- Cycles of cramping pain about every 15-30 minutes that cause the child to cry and pull knees to chest.
- Distended painful abdomen.
- Diarrhea, bloody stools, or no stools.
- Vomiting (occurring soon after crying begins usually indicates small intestine obstruction; later vomiting usually indicated large intestine blockage)
- Tachycardia and tachypnea.
- Decreased urinary output.
- Fever.

Treatment includes:

- Surgical repair (Ladd procedure) is indicated immediately if there is volvulus and most malrotations require surgical repair even with less severe symptoms.

Intussusception

Intussusception is a telescoping of one portion of the intestine into another, usually at the ileocecal valve, causing an obstruction. As the walls of the intestine come in contact, inflammation and edema cause decreased perfusion, which can result in infarction with peritonitis and death. Fecal material cannot move past the obstruction. It is most common between 3-12 months but can occur until 6 years and may relate to viral infections. **Symptoms** include:

- "Current jelly stool" composed of blood and mucous (occurs with 60%).
- Sudden acute episodes of severe abdominal pain during which child pulls knees to chest.
- Vomiting.
- Lethargy and weakness.
- Distended abdomen, painful to palpation.
- Sausage-shaped mass in RUQ of abdomen.
- Progressive fever and prostration if peritonitis occurs.

Treatment includes:

- Barium or air enema to diagnose and apply pressure that may resolve the intussusception.
- Surgical repair if there is shock, peritonitis, intestinal perforation, or failure to resolve with barium/air enema.

GER

Gastroesophageal reflux (GER) *is* involuntary regurgitation of stomach contents into the esophagus, usually caused by decreased tone in the lower esophageal sphincter in children. GER **symptoms** include:

- *Infants:* Frequent regurgitation, especially after feeding, usually not associated with respiratory distress although some children may have colicky symptoms.
- *Toddler/older children:* Less obvious regurgitation because they are upright more and eat solid foods, but they may refuse food or indicate or complain of pain in epigastric region. They may exhibit failure to thrive or weight loss, asthma, cough, or pneumonia from aspiration of gastric fluids.

Treatment includes:

- Regulating feeding to avoid over-feeding and (for older children) avoiding large meals or after dinner snacking.
- Positioning: prone positioning after feeding/eating reduces regurgitation (although some concern remains about SIDS with infants). Placing infant in an upright position (avoiding slumping) after meals or carrying the infant upright can help.
- Medications: Histamine-2 receptor blockers and/or antacids (without aluminum).

NEC

Necrotizing enterocolitis is an inflammatory bowel disease affecting primarily preterm/premature infants, characterized by an immature bowel that has suffered a hypoxic episode with resultant inflammation and necrosis of the intestinal wall, allowing gas into tissues of the wall, the portal venous system, and/or peritoneal cavity. It may result in infarction and/or perforation. The distal ileum and proximal colon are most-commonly affected. The cause is not clearly understood, but appears related to an ischemic episode, colonization by bacteria, and excess/rapid enteral feedings. Mortality rates are about 30%.

Symptoms include:

- Gastric retention/ abdominal distention.
- Periods of apnea.
- Vomiting (bilious).
- Occult or frank blood (25%) in stool.
- Pneumatosis intestinalis (gas in intestinal wall) (75%)
- Portal venous gas (10-30%).
- Decrease in urinary output.
- Jaundice.
- Unstable temperature.

Treatment includes:

- Cessation of oral feeding.
- NG decompression.
- Systemic antibiotics.
- Correcting fluid and electrolyte imbalance.
- Surgical repair with bowel resection may be necessary.

Hirschsprung's Disease

Hirschsprung's disease (congenital aganglionic megacolon) is failure of ganglion nerve cells to migrate to part of the bowel (usually the distal colon), so that part of the bowel lacks enervation and peristalsis, causing stool to accumulate and leading to distention and megacolon. There is a genetic predisposition to the disease that affects more males than females and is associated with trisomy 21 (Down syndrome). **Symptoms** include:

- Failure to pass meconium in 24-48 hours.
- Poor feeding. Bilious vomitus. Abdominal distention.

Delayed diagnosis:

- Chronic constipation. Failure to thrive.
- Periods of diarrhea and vomiting.
- (With infection) Severe prostration with watery diarrhea, fever, hypotension.

Childhood symptoms:

- Chronic constipation with ribbon-like stools.
- Abdominal distention with visible peristalsis and palpable fecal mass. Poorly-nourished, anemic, child.

Treatment includes:

- Resection of aganglionic section and colorectal anastomosis. There are a number of procedures (Swenson, Duhamel, and Soave) but recently laparoscopic or trans-anal minimally-invasive approaches have proven successful.

Abdominal Wall Malrotation Defect

Umbilical Hernia

Umbilical hernia is a skin-covered herniation of intestine and omentum through an abdominal wall defect near the umbilicus caused by an incomplete closure of the umbilical ring. The herniation may range from 1-5 cm in size and may be obvious on physical examination or felt on palpation. It may appear flat when the child is supine but protrude when the child is upright or crying. Approximately 1 in 6 infants are born with umbilical hernias. Symptoms are usually absent unless strangulation of the hernia occurs, and then the infant may cry with pain, feed poorly, vomit, and have an increase in temperature. The abdomen may become distended. In this case, emergency surgical repair must be done. Treatment usually involves just observing the hernia for complications as, in most cases, it will reduce on its own. If the hernia is still present at 3-4 years, a simple surgical repair of the hernia may be done.

Congenital Diaphragmatic Hernia

Congenital diaphragmatic hernia is herniation of abdominal contents into chest cavity. During fetal development, a hole in the diaphragm that should close at about 3 months stays open, allowing loops of the intestine or the stomach to herniate into the chest and preventing adequate development of the lungs (pulmonary hypoplasia) and/or heart. The infants are usually very dyspneic at birth and may need to be ventilated. They may need temporary heart/bypass as well. The kidneys are often enlarged. Radiographic studies are done to show the extent of the abnormality, usually showing a high gastrointestinal obstruction, often at the duodenum. A nasogastric feeding tube is inserted and an intravenous line. Supportive treatment is given for dyspnea as well as correction of acidosis. Surgical repair may be done after birth or delayed for weeks until child stabilizes. Surgical repair may be done in one stage or more, depending upon the degree of abnormality.

Hernia Repair

Hernia repair (herniorrhaphy) is the most common surgery for infants and children and is done to repair herniation of the peritoneum and a segment of bowel through the abdominal wall. Surgery is necessary to prevent an incarcerated hernia, in which the bowel twists and blood supply is compromised. There are 3 main types:

- *Inguinal:* Herniation in the inguinal canal. This is common in premature or low birth-weight infants, usually males, and may occur bilaterally.
- *Femoral:* Herniation posterior to the inguinal ligament. This is more common in females.
- *Umbilical:* Herniation in the umbilical ring.

Inguinal and femoral hernias are usually repaired as soon as possible because of the danger of incarceration; however, umbilical hernias pose less concern and often heal over time without surgical repair, so it is rarely done prior to school age. If incarceration has occurred prior to surgery, the affected segment of bowel is resected. Surgery may be done laparoscopically.

Encopresis and Fecal Incontinence

Encopresis is the voluntary or involuntary passage of stool in places or manners that are inappropriate for a child, 80% of whom are male, 4 years or older. There are two types: retentive encopresis, which accounts for about 80% of those affected, and non-retentive, which accounts for the other 20%. Retentive encopresis is characterized by a history of long term, painful constipation and the development of overflow diarrhea. The chronic constipation causes distention of the rectum and stretching of both the internal and external anal sphincters; as a result, the child may no longer feel the urge to defecate, so stool eventually leaks from the rectum, causing chronic fecal incontinence. Non-retentive encopresis, usually involving passage of normally formed stools on a daily basis, does not involve constipation or bowel abnormalities, except in a small subset that may have irritable bowel syndrome, but is generally a behavioral/psychological problem.

Constipation and Impaction

Constipation is a condition with bowel movements less frequent than normal for a child, or hard, small stool that is evacuated fewer than 3 times weekly. Food moves through the gastrointestinal from the small intestine to the colon in semi-liquid form. Constipation results from the colon, where fluid is absorbed. If too much fluid is absorbed, the stool can become too dry. Children may have abdominal distention and cramps and need to strain for defecation.

Fecal impaction occurs when the hard stool moves into the rectum and becomes a large, dense, immovable mass that cannot be evacuated even with straining, usually as a result of chronic constipation. In addition to abdominal cramps and distention, the person may feel intense rectal pressure and pain accompanied by a sense of urgency to defecate. Nausea and vomiting may also occur. Fecal incontinence, with liquid stool leaking about the impaction is common. Constipation in small children is most common between 2-4 and may be associated with diet or toilet training.

Management Strategies

Management strategies for constipation and impaction include:

- *Add fiber* with bran, fresh/dried fruits, and whole grains,
- *Increase fluids* (other than milk, which is constipating) according to age.

Increased physical activity

- *Change in medications* causing constipation.
- *Stool softeners,* such as Colace®, or bulk formers, such as Metamucil®, may decrease fluid absorption and move stool through the colon more quickly.
- *Laxatives,* such as milk of magnesia or polyethylene glycol (PEG) may be used occasionally, but overuse of laxatives can cause constipation.
- *Delayed toileting* should be avoided and bowel training regimen done to promote evacuation at the same time each day. Toilet sitting should begin 3-4 times daily for 10 minutes, decreasing to 2 times daily for 10 minutes.
- *Enemas, laxatives, and manual removal of impaction* may be necessary initially, depending upon the severity of the constipation/impaction, but should not be given by parents.

Diarrhea

Diarrhea is common in infants and children and can be caused by a variety of different infections and conditions. Diarrhea accounts for about 20% of hospitalizations of children <2 and causes about 500 deaths in children <4 in the United States each year. Because of the potential for loss of fluids, electrolytes, and nutrition, and the danger of ulceration and bleeding, diarrhea should be monitored carefully to determine the **cause**:

- *Osmotic*: Increased fluid in the stool and may be related to lactose intolerance and overfeeding.
- *Secretory*: Inhibited electrolyte (ion) absorption or increased electrolyte secretion related to bacterial endotoxins.
- *Motility disorders*: Interfere with absorption of fluids, including bile salt or pancreatic enzyme deficiencies.
- *Inflammatory*: Related to Crohn's disease or ulcerative colitis.

Viral/bacterial: The most common cause of diarrhea in children. A wide range of viral and bacterial pathogens can cause mild to severe life-threatening diarrhea.

Bacterial Infections

A wide range of bacterial and viral pathogens can cause mild to severe life-threatening diarrhea:

- *Campylobacter jejuni* transmitted from pets to children <7 through contaminated food and water, usually in the summer. Diarrhea with fever, vomiting, and abdominal pain persists 7-12 days. *Treatment:* Erythromycin (40 mg/kg/day) in 3 doses daily for 5-7 days.
- *Clostridium difficile* occurs secondary to antibiotic use. Some children are asymptomatic carriers, but severe illness is life threatening with bloody diarrhea and abdominal pain leading to megacolon. *Treatment:* Metronidazole 30mg/kg/day in 4 doses or Vancomycin 40mg/kg/day in 4 doses for 7-10 days.
- *Yersinia enterocolitica* found in uncooked pork or unpasteurized milk causes secretory diarrhea in all ages with fever, foul, green and bloody stool, and pain in right lower abdomen. Usually resolves in 3-4 days.

- *Shigella* is transmitted fecal-oral route from contaminated food and water and occurs from 6-36 months. Characterized by bloody diarrhea, abdominal pain, and fever. *Treatment:* TMP-SMZ 8 mg TMP/kg/day in 2 doses for 7-10 days.

Salmonella

Salmonella causes up to 4 million infections in the United States, resulting in 500 deaths, primarily of young children. *Salmonella* is spread by the fecal-oral route through ingestion of contaminated food or water, including all meats, milk, eggs, and vegetables. Raw or undercooked meat, unpasteurized milk, and unwashed produce are high-risk. *Salmonella* may be found in the feces of pets, particularly reptiles such as snakes and turtles. Small children should not have reptiles as pets. **Symptoms** appear 12-72 hours after infection and include bloody diarrhea with abdominal pain, fever, and vomiting. Most cases resolve within 7-10 days, but in some cases, life-threatening sepsis may occur, requiring **treatment** with antibiotics. Amoxicillin 40 g/kg/day in 3 doses for 7-10 days is the antibiotic of choice. Antibiotic prophylaxis is usually contraindicated except in children <1 year that are at risk for bacteremia or those who are immunocompromised.

Escherichia coli

Escherichia coli is part of the normal flora of the intestines and serves to inhibit other bacteria, but 5 serotypes can cause intestinal disease and severe diarrhea. Some types are more common in developing countries and may occur in children who are traveling in areas where feces have contaminated food supplies and water. Severe outbreaks of *E. coli* infection have occurred in the United States with a toxic strain, O157:H7, which produces a toxin that can cause damage to the intestinal lining, including blood vessels, resulting in hemorrhage and watery diarrhea that becomes bloody. This hemorrhagic colitis usually clears with supportive treatment after 10 days. However, about 15% of children develop sepsis and hemolytic uremic syndrome with kidney failure, hemolytic anemia, and thrombocytopenia. Death rates are 3-5%, but residual renal and neurological damage may result. **Treatment** is supportive with intravenous therapy, blood transfusions, and kidney dialysis. Antibiotics and antidiarrheals are contraindicated as they may worsen *E. coli* infections.

Intestinal Parasites

Giardia Lamblia

Giardia lamblia is a protozoan that infects water supplies and spreads to children through the fecal-oral route. It is the most common cause of non-bacterial diarrhea in the United States, causing about 20,000 cases of infection each year in all ages. Children often become infected by swallowing recreational waters (pools, lakes) while swimming or putting contaminated items into the mouth. *Giardia* live and multiply within the small intestine where cysts develop. **Symptoms** occur 7-14 days after ingestion of 1 or more cysts and include: diarrhea with greasy floating stools (rarely bloody), stomach cramps, nausea, and flatulence, lasting 2-6 weeks. A chronic infection may develop that can last for months or years. **Treatment** includes: Furazolidone 5-8mg/kg/day in 4 doses for 7-10 days or Metronidazole 40mg/kg/day in 3 doses for 7-10 days. Chronic infections are often very resistant to treatment.

Roundworms

Worldwide, there are numerous helminths (worms) that can cause intestinal infections. Studies estimate that 50 million children in the United States are infected with worms. Risk factors include:

- Young age.
- Going barefoot.
- Poor sanitation of food and water.
- Poor hygiene.
- Living in or traveling to an endemic area.
- Immigrant status, especially from Mexico.

Roundworms (Ascaris lumbricoides) can grow 6-13 inches in length, and a child may have up to 100 worms. After ingestion of eggs from contaminated raw foods or vegetables, the worms migrate to the intestines but can migrate to other organs, such as the lungs, and cause serious damage. They may also multiply in clumps and cause intestinal obstruction or may penetrate the intestinal wall causing peritonitis. *Symptoms* include malnutrition, abdominal discomfort, and passing worms in stool or emesis. *Treatment* includes: Pyrantel pamoate 11 mg/kg in one dose or Mebendazole 100mg times 3 days. Piperazine citrate 75mg/kg/day for 2 days for intestinal obstruction.

Enterobius Vermicularis (Pinworms)

Enterobius vermicularis (pinworms) are tiny (3-13 mm) worms that hatch in the small intestine after ingestion of eggs. The mature worms crawl through the rectum to lay eggs in the perianal folds, causing intense itching, often resulting in repeat self-infection as the child scratches and then touches the hand to the mouth or contaminates food. Infection may result from contact with contaminated surfaces as well. The larvae hatch in the small intestines, but the adults live in the colon. Pinworms are the most common helminthic infection in the United States, affecting about 40 million people, especially children. Many are asymptomatic except for intense perianal itching although some may have abdominal discomfort and anorexia or develop secondary infections from scratching. Girls may develop vulvovaginitis from invasion of the genital tract. Diagnosis is made by the "scotch tape" test or anal swabs. **Treatment** includes: Mebendazole 100mg for one dose repeated in 2 weeks or Pyrantel pamoate 11mg/kg for 1 dose repeated in 2 weeks.

Necator Americanus (Hookworms)

Necator americanus is the most common species of hookworm found in the southeastern United States. Hookworm larvae may be swallowed directly or penetrate the skin, often the feet of children going barefoot, and migrate to the lungs where they are coughed up and swallowed and carried to the small intestines where they attach themselves to the walls to suck blood and multiply. Severe infection can result in hypochromic, microcytic anemia along with hypoproteinemia and malnutrition. Infection with hookworms can result in dyspnea, cardiomegaly, and arrhythmias and can be fatal in infants. Infected children may have restricted growth and mental development, which may be irreversible. Diagnosis is with serial stool specimens.

Symptoms include itching and rash at the site of infection, followed by abdominal pain, diarrhea, anorexia, weight loss, and anemia.

Treatment includes: Mebendazole 100mg times 3 days. Iron supplements may be necessary. Stools must be rechecked 1 week after treatment so that repeat treatment can be done if needed.

Crohn's Disease

Crohn's disease manifests with inflammation of the GI system. Inflammation is transmural (often leading to intestinal stenosis and fistulas), focal and discontinuous with aphthous ulcerations progressing to linear and irregular shaped ulcerations. Granulomas may be present. Common sites of inflammation are the terminal ileum and cecum. Condition is usually chronic, but an acute flare-up may mimic appendicitis. Children may have delayed development and stunted growth. There is a genetic component to the disease.

Symptoms include:

- Perirectal abscess/fistula in advanced disease.
- *Diarrhea* is usually present with colonic disease. May have nocturnal bowel movements, watery stools, and rectal hemorrhage.
- *Anemia* may develop with chronic bleeding.
- *Abdominal pain* most common in lower right quadrant, usually indicating transmural inflammation; may include post-prandial pain and cramping,

Other symptoms include nausea and vomiting (usually related to strictures of small intestine), weight loss (with small intestine involvement), fever, and night sweats. **Treatment** includes:

- Corticosteroids and antibiotics for acute exacerbations.
- Immunomodulatory agents (cyclosporine, methotrexate).
- Antidiarrheals.
- Aminosalicylates.

Ulcerative Colitis

Ulcerative colitis is superficial inflammation of mucosa of colon and rectum, causing ulcerations in the areas where inflammation has destroyed cells. These ulcerations, ranging from pinpoint to extensive, may bleed and produce purulent material. The mucosa of the bowel becomes swollen, erythematous, and granular. Onset is usually between ages 15 and 30, and there is a genetic component. Ulcerative colitis may affect only the rectum (ulcerative proctitis), the entire colon (pancolitis), or only the left colon (limited or distal colitis).

Symptoms include:

- Abdominal pain may be absent or mild unless severe disease.
- Bloody diarrhea/rectal bleeding in absence of infection may result in anemia and fluid and electrolyte depletion. Diarrhea more frequent as colonic involvement increases.
- Fecal urgency and tenesmus may occur.
- Anorexia resulting in weight loss, fatigue.
- Systemic disorders with eye inflammation, arthritis, liver disease, and osteoporosis as immune system triggers generalized inflammation.

Treatment includes:

- Aminosalicylates
- Steroids
- Immunomodulatory agents
- Antispasmodics
- Iron supplementation
- High-protein diet with decreased fiber

Familial Adenomatous Polyposis

Familial adenomatous polyposis (FAP) is an inherited autosomal-dominant syndrome where people develop hundreds to thousands of colorectal polyps between ages 5-40 with cancer usually in one or multiple polyps by about age 20. Between 20-40, virtually everyone develops cancer. A genetic factor predisposes people with this genetic mutation to other malignancies, especially in duodenum and stomach. They may develop *Gardner syndrome* with congenital hypertrophy of retinal pigment (CHRP), sebaceous cysts, desmoid tumors (fibrous tumors arising in tissue covering intestines), and benign bone tumors. Identifying FAP before colorectal cancer develops is critical as prophylactic colectomy may be indicated with high risk. People with familial history of FAP should have genetic testing.

Variant forms of FAP are as follows:

- *Attenuated familial adenomatous polyposis* has delayed *polyp* growth, with onset of colorectal cancer at about 55 years of age.
- *Autosomal recessive familial adenomatous polyposis* typically causes fewer than 100 polyps and is caused by mutation on different gene than other forms.

Peptic Ulcer Disease

Peptic ulcer disease (PUD) includes both ulcerations of the duodenum and stomach. They may be primary (usually duodenal) or secondary (usually gastric). Gastric ulcers are commonly associated with cytomegalovirus and *Helicobacter pylori* infections in children. *H. pylori* is spread in the fecal-oral route from person to person or contaminated water and causes a chronic inflammation and ulcerations of the gastric mucosa. PUD is 2-3 times more common in males and is associated with poor economic status resulting in a crowded unhygienic environment although it can occur in other children. Usually others in the family have a history of ulcers as well. *Symptoms* include abdominal pain, nausea, vomiting and GI bleeding in children <6 with epigastric and post-prandial pain and indigestion in older children. **Treatment** includes:

- Antibiotics for *H. pylori*: Amoxicillin, Clarithromycin, Metronidazole.
- Proton pump inhibitors: Lansoprazole or omeprazole.
- Sucralfate.
- Histamine-receptor antagonists: Cimetidine, ranitidine, famotidine.

Infantile Colic

Infantile colic is a disorder that causes severe intestinal cramping in infants <3 months old, accompanied by severe bouts of crying, often unrelieved by comfort measures. Colic may persist in some children beyond 3 months. Typical **diagnostic pattern** is >3 hours crying, 3 days a week for >3 weeks. Occurrence rates vary because of different definitions that range from 5-40%. The cause is unknown but may relate to rapid feeding, sensitivity to formula, swallowing excessive air during feeding, cigarette smoke in the environment, inadequate burping after feeding. **Treatment** requires observation of feeding to determine proper feeding and providing support and encouragement to the mother. Various comfort measures work with different infants: driving in a car, sitting in a vibrating seat, swaddling the infant, and applying firm pressure to the abdomen. Parent should keep a journal that notes feeding times and crying times to help establish patterns to assist in diagnosis and ruling out of other causes for symptoms.

Imperforate Anus

Imperforate anus (anorectal malfunction) is a congenital abnormality where the rectum is absent, malformed, or displaced from normal position. It may include disorders of the urinary tract. Imperforate anus occurs in 1 in 5000 births, more commonly in males than females. Imperforate anus may include stenosis or atresia of anus. There are 3 main categories, classified according to relationship of rectum to puborectalis musculature:

- *Low anomalies:* No external opening, but rectum is otherwise in normal position through the puborectalis muscle, with normal function, and no connection to the genitourinary tract.
- *Intermediate anomalies:* Rectum is at or below the level of puborectalis muscle and an anal dimple is evident. The external sphincter is in normal position.
- *High anomalies:* Rectum ends above the puborectalis muscles, and internal sphincter is absent. Frequently, there is a rectourethral fistula in males or a rectovaginal fistula in females. There may be fistulas to the bladder or perineum.

Symptoms are as follows:

- *Absence of anal opening:* No meconium in 24-48 hours, abdominal distention, and vomiting.
- *Rectovaginal fistula or rectourethral fistula:* Symptoms may not be evident at first because stool passes through fistula.
- *Fistula between the rectum and the bladder:* Gas or fecal material may be expelled per the urethra. *Displacement of the anus:* Chronic constipation develops over time.

Diagnosis is as follows:

- Physical examination. Digital or endoscopic examination.
- *Contrast radiography* with the infant inverted and an opaque marker at the anal dimple will outline the location of a pouch in relation to the normal position of the anus.

Most forms of imperforate anus require **treatment** by surgery, type depending upon extent of abnormality:

- *Simple excision* of anal opening may suffice.
- *2-3 step procedures* for higher anomalies in which a colostomy is first performed with later reconstruction of the anus in the proper position, involving anoplasty and pull through procedures.
- *Manual dilation* may treat stenosis.

Review of Systems: Cardiovascular

Normal Fetal Blood Circulation

Fetal blood circulation begins with oxygenated blood in the umbilical cord flowing through the umbilicus with half to the liver and the other half to the *ductus venosus* vessel, carrying blood to the inferior vena cava where it mixes with deoxygenated blood and flows to the vena cava and right atrium. With non-functioning lungs, most blood bypasses the right ventricle, and the blood shunts directly from the right to the left atrium through the *foramen ovale*, a small opening with a valve, the *septum primum*, to prevent backflow, and to the ascending aorta and cranial arteries. A small amount of deoxygenated blood from the superior vena cava circulates through the pulmonary trunk, but most of this deoxygenated blood bypasses the lungs and enters the *ductus arteriosus*, connecting the pulmonary trunk to the descending aortic arch, where there is both oxygenated and deoxygenated blood, some of which will circulate to the lower body and some into the umbilical arteries to return to the placenta for reoxygenation.

Normal Cardiac Rates for Infants and Children

Normal cardiac rates can vary widely from one child to another, so it's important to understand the normal range in order to determine if the child has an abnormal pulse. They will also vary depending upon whether the child is awake, sleeping, or active. Pulse rate should be taken with a stethoscope, especially for infants and small children, as the pulse may be difficult to palpate or count accurately manually. This allows assessment for murmurs.

- **Newborn infant:**
  - At rest: 100-180
  - Asleep: 80-160
  - Active/sick: ≤ 220
- **1-12 weeks:**
  - At rest: 100-220
  - Asleep: 80-200
  - Active/sick: ≤ 220
- **3-24 months:**
  - At rest: 80-150
  - Asleep: 70-120
  - Active/sick: ≤ 200
- **2-10 years:**
  - At rest: 70-110
  - Asleep: 60-90
  - Active/sick: ≤ 200
- **10 years to adult:**
  - At rest: 55-90
  - Asleep: 50-90
  - Active/sick: ≤ 200

Normal Conduction of the Heart

The normal **conduction of the heart** has 4 stages:

1. *Generation of impulse at the Sino-atrial (SA) node* (primary pacemaker) located at the junction of the right atrium and superior vena cava. The electrical impulse travels cells of the atria along internodal pathways, causing electrical stimulation and contraction of the atria.
2. *Atrioventricular node conduction of impulse.* This occurs when the impulses from the SA node reach the AV node in the right atrial wall near the tricuspid valve. There is a slight delay (about one-tenth of a second), allowing the atria to empty.
3. *Atrioventricular bundle (bundle of His) conduction.* The AV node relays the impulse to the ventricles through the atrioventricular bundle; specialized conduction cells in the ventricular septum that branch to the right and left ventricles, carrying the electrical impulse.
4. *Purkinje Fiber conduction.* The impulses are conducted down the AV bundles to the base of the heart where they divide into Purkinje fibers, which stimulate the myocardial cells to contract the ventricles.

Congestive Heart Failure

Congestive heart failure is a symptom rather than a disease. It results from the inability of the heart to adequately pump the blood that is needed for the body. In children (primarily infants) it most often occurs secondary to cardiac abnormalities with resultant increased blood volume and blood pressure:

- *Right-sided failure* occurs if the right ventricle cannot effectively contract to pump blood into the pulmonary artery, causing pressure to build in the right atrium and the venous circulation. This venous hypertension can result in peripheral edema or ascites and hepatosplenomegaly.
- *Left-sided failure* occurs if the left ventricle cannot effectively pump blood into the aorta and systemic circulation, increasing pressure in the left atrium and the pulmonary veins, with resultant pulmonary edema and increased pulmonary pressure.

Children often have some combination of both right and left-sided failure, depending on their cardiac defect.

Symptoms in Infants and Children

Congestive heart failure symptoms vary widely depending upon the type and degree the primary cause, and the child's age. Because of increased pressure in the lungs after birth, symptoms may be delayed in infants for the first week or two:

- *Infants* with left failure typically suffer respiratory distress with tachypnea, grunting respirations, sternal retraction, and rales, but the most common symptom is failure to thrive and difficulty eating, often leaving the child exhausted and sweaty. Those with right-sided failure may have more generalized edema of lower extremities, distended abdomen from ascites, hepatomegaly and jugular venous distension. Tachycardia and low cardiac output occur with both types of heart failure resulting in sweating, pallor, and hypotension.

- *Older children* typically suffer from inability to tolerate activity or exercise, becoming short of breath on exertion. Appetite is often poor with weight loss.
- In *adolescents,* CHF may be caused by the use of illicit drugs if there is no structural or acquired heart disease.

Management in Infants and Children

Management of congestive heart failure (CHF) in infants and children can be difficult. It is extremely important to establish the etiology and to treat the underlying cause. For infants with structural cardiac abnormalities, surgical repair may be needed to resolve the CHF. There are some medical treatments that can relieve **symptoms**:

- *Diuretics,* such as furosemide (Lasix®), metolazone, or hydrochlorothiazide to reduce pulmonary and peripheral edema.
- *Antihypertensives,* such as Captopril® or Propranolol® to decrease heart workload.
- *Cardiac glycosides,* such as Lanoxin®, may relieve symptoms if above medicines are not successful.
- *High caloric feedings,* either by bottle or nasogastric feeding to provide sufficient nutrients.
- *Oxygen* may be useful for some children with weak hearts.
- *Restriction of activities* to reduce stress on the heart.
- *Dopamine or dobutamine* may be given to increase the contractibility of the heart.

Chronic and Acute Heart Failure

Chronic heart failure develops more slowly with the myocardium damaged by lack of adequate oxygenation and nutrition, so that the myocardial cells begin to die, creating areas of necrosis, which in turn stimulates the production of fibroblasts, which replace cells with deposits of collagen, creating a fibrotic resistant myocardium. Existing myocytes increase in size but lose strength. There is cardiac dilation and increasing vascular resistance (afterload).

Acute heart failure can occur with sudden onset, with the body attempting to compensate for circulatory malfunction by protecting blood flow to vital organs. There is an increase in the contractibility of the myocardium but peripheral vasoconstriction. Fluid and sodium are retained to control hypotension. However, the increased contractibility and heart rate increases the need for oxygen beyond that available, leading to physiologic response that result in tissue necrosis, cardiotoxicity, pulmonary edema, and organ failure.

- *Capillary hypertension* decreases oncotic pressure and results in vasodilation and increased loss of fluid from the plasma to the interstitial fluid, resulting in pulmonary edema.
- *Capillary hypotension* results in increased oncotic pressure and pulls fluid back into the plasma, a result of shock.

Cardiac-Related Pulmonary Edema

Pulmonary edema occurs when excess fluid enters the pulmonary interstitium and alveoli because of increased pulmonary capillary pressure combined with decrease in the oncotic pressure, mechanical or physiologic damage to the capillary-alveolar membrane, or obstruction of the lymphatic drainage system:

- Mitral stenosis reduces the flow of blood to the left ventricle. Pressure in the left atrium increases to overcome resistance, resulting in enlargement of the left atrium and increased pressure in the pulmonary veins and capillaries of the lung.

91

- Tachycardia and/or atrial fibrillation may reduce blood flow to the left ventricle, resulting in increased atrial and pulmonary pressure.
- Left ventricular dysfunction reduces cardiac output and fluid backs up into the lungs, increasing the capillary pressure.

The increased pressure results in increased capillary vasodilation and fluid flows into the interstitium. Initially, lymphatic drainage increases to compensate but becomes overwhelmed as fluid accumulates. When the interstitium becomes engorged, the fluid crosses the alveolar membranes, and the alveoli cannot function, resulting in decreased gas exchange and hypoxemia.

Myocarditis

Myocarditis is inflammation of the cardiac myocardium (muscle tissue), usually triggered by a viral infection, such as the Influenza virus, Coxsackie virus, and HIV. It can also be caused by bacteria, fungi, or parasites. In some cases, it is also a complication of endocarditis. It may also be triggered by chemotherapy drugs and some antibiotics. One problem with children is that the immune response against the invading organism may be overly aggressive, invading the heart muscle and producing toxins that damage cells and cause further damage to the heart muscle. Myocarditis can result in dilation of the heart, development of thrombi on the heart walls (known as mural thrombi), infiltration of blood cells around the coronary vessels and between muscle fibers, causing further degeneration of the muscle tissue. The heart may become enlarged and weak, as the ability to pump blood is impaired, leading to congestive heart failure.

Diagnosis and Treatment

Diagnosis of myocarditis depends upon the clinical picture, as there is no test specific for myocarditis although a number of tests may be done to verify the clinical diagnosis:

- *Chest radiograph* may indicate cardiomegaly or pulmonary edema.
- *EKG* may show non-specific changes.
- *Echocardiogram* may indicate cardiomegaly and demonstrate defects in functioning.
- *Cardiac catheterization* and cardiac biopsy will yield confirmation in 65% of cases, but not all of the heart muscle may be affected, so a negative finding does not rule out myocarditis.
- *Viral cultures* of nasopharynx and rectal may help to identify organism.
- *Viral titers* may increase as disease progresses.
- *Polymerase chain reaction (PCR)* of biopsy specimen may be most effective for diagnosis.

Treatment aims to hemodynamic needs and maintain tissue perfusion:

- Restriction of activities.
- *Careful monitoring* for heart failure and medical treatment as indicated (diuretics, digoxin, etc.)
- *Oxygen* as needed to maintain normal oxygen saturation.
- *IV gamma globulin* for acute stage.

Pericarditis

Pericarditis is inflammation of the pericardial membrane that surrounds the heart. The outer fibrous pericardium is connective tissue that is continuous with the outer layers of the great vessels and serves to protect and anchor the heart. The inner serous pericardium has two layers separated with serous pericardial fluid to lubricate the heart and prevent friction. With pericarditis, the layers may become attached to each other (dry), or the serous fluid may be replaced by purulent material,

92

calcifications, fibrinous material, or blood. Pericarditis is frequently associated with surgical repair of cardiac structural abnormalities, but it may also result from other systemic viral, bacterial, fungal, or parasitic infections or may be caused by direct trauma. Some chronic connective tissue disorders, such as lupus erythematosus, may also cause pericarditis. Pericarditis is often accompanied by fever, dysrhythmia, poor appetite, irritability, malaise, and sharp piercing chest pain.

Medical Management

Pericarditis is treated according to the cause and the type and extent of inflammation as well as the age, size, and condition of the child. Diagnostic procedures are similar to those for endocarditis and myocarditis. **Treatment** includes:

- *Analgesics* as indicated to control pain.
- *Anti-inflammatory drugs*, aspirin or ibuprofen, may be used to relieve discomfort and increase the rate of fluid reabsorption.
- *Restriction of activity* is necessary if cardiac function and output is impaired.
- *Corticosteroids* are used in some cases if there is no response to anti-inflammatory drugs.
- *Surgical intervention* may include pericardiocentesis, which is removing fluid from the pericardial sac in order to relieve increasing pressure and to diagnose the causative agent. In some cases, a small opening may be made into the pericardium to allow continuous drainage of exudate into the chest cavity. In severe cases, the outer layer of the pericardium may need to be removed if it is preventing functioning of the ventricles.

Cardiac Hypertrophy

Cardiac hypertrophy occurs when the heart responds to stresses, such as an increase in blood pressure or structural abnormality that interferes with normal functioning, by adapting its size and shape according to the increased effort required to function. As the heart adapts, the heart muscle enlarges, but this change is not the result of proliferation of cells but an increase in the size of existing myocytes (muscles cells). Thus, the cells are not dividing and providing more cells but simply getting bigger, and sometimes crowding out and killing other cells, further increasing the stress on the heart and again causing the cells to enlarge in a cycle that progressively weakens the musculature or the heart. Recent studies show 12% of children with HIV demonstrate cardiac hypertrophy, and 55% of children with renal transplants showed left ventricular hypertrophy, suggesting that many of these children are at risk for congestive heart failure. Treating the cause of hypertrophy does not always reduce the hypertrophic changes.

Hypertrophic Cardiomyopathy

Hypertrophic cardiomyopathy (also known as asymmetric septal hypertrophy) is a rare genetic and occasionally idiopathic disorder that is often undetected until adolescence when the increasing symptoms become noticeable. With hypertrophic cardiomyopathy, the heart mass and size increase, especially with thickness along the septum, resulting in smaller ventricular capacity so that the ventricles fill less efficiently and the atria have to work harder. This thickening may be asymmetrical. The disease may be nonobstructive or obstructive. The increased size of the septum may pull structures, such as the mitral valve, out of alignment, causing some obstruction of the flow of blood through the valve to the aorta (idiopathic hypertrophic subaortic stenosis). The changes in the ventricles may result in increasing diastolic abnormalities although systolic function is usually normal or high. When diagnosed in young people, the disease is often more severe than in those who are diagnosed later in life.

Acyanotic and Cyanotic Congenital Heart Disease

Congenital heart disease is one of the leading causes of death in children within the first year of life. There are two main types of congenital heart disease: acyanotic and cyanotic. **Acyanotic defects** include those with increased pulmonary blood flow or obstructed ventricular blood flow.

- **Increased pulmonary blood flow:**
  - *Atrial septal defect*
  - *Atrioventricular canal defect*
  - *Patent ductus arteriosus*
  - *Ventricular septal defect*
- **Obstructed ventricular blood flow:**
  - *Aortic stenosis*
  - *Coarctation of aorta*
  - *Pulmonic stenosis*
  - *Cyanotic congenital heart disease includes those with decreased pulmonary blood flow and mixed blood flow.*
- **Decreased pulmonary blood flow:**
  - *Tetralogy of Fallot*
  - *Tricuspid atresia*
- **Mixed blood flow:**
  - *Hypoplastic left heart syndrome*
  - *Total anomalous pulmonary venous return*
  - *Transposition of great arteries*
  - *Truncus arteriosus*

Atrioventricular Canal Defect

Atrioventricular canal defect is often associated with Down syndrome and involves a number of different defects, including openings between the atria and ventricles as well as abnormalities of the valves. In partial defects, there is an opening between the atria and mitral valve regurgitation. In complete defects, there is a large central hole in the heart and only one common valve between the atria and ventricles. The blood may flow freely about the heart, usually from left to right. Extra blood flow to the lungs causes enlargement of the heart. Partial defects may go undiagnosed for 20 years. **Symptoms** include:

- Typical congestive heart failure signs:
  - Weakness and fatigue.
  - Cough and/or wheezing with production of white or bloody sputum.
  - Peripheral edema and ascites.
  - Dysrhythmia and tachycardia.
- Dyspnea
- Poor appetite
- Failure to thrive, low weight
- Cyanosis of skin and lips.

Treatment includes:

- Open-heart surgery to patch holes in the septum and valve repair or replacement.

Atrial Septal Defect

An **atrial septal defect (ASD)** is an abnormal opening in the septum between the right and left atria. Because the left atrium has higher pressure than the right atrium, some of the oxygenated blood returning from the lungs to the left atrium is shunted back to the right atrium where it is again returned to the lungs, displacing deoxygenated blood. **Symptoms** may be few, depending upon the degree of the defect but can include:

- Asymptomatic (some infants).
- Congestive heart failure.
- Heart murmur.
- Increased risk for dysrhythmias and pulmonary vascular obstructive disease over time

Treatment may not be necessary for small defects, but larger defects require closure:

- Open-heart surgical repair may be done.
- Heart catheterization and placing of closure device (Amplatz® device) across the atrial septal defect.

Ventricular Septal Defect

Ventricular septal defect is an abnormal opening in the septum between the right and left ventricles. If the opening is small, the child may be asymptomatic, but larger openings can result in a left to right shunt because of higher pressure in the left ventricle. This shunting increases over 6 weeks after birth with symptoms becoming more evident, but the defect may close within a few years. **Symptoms** may include:

- Congestive heart failure with peripheral edema.
- Tachycardia.
- Dyspnea.
- Difficulty feeding.
- Heart murmur.
- Recurrent pulmonary infections.
- Increased risk for bacterial endocarditis and pulmonary vascular obstructive disease.

Treatment includes:

- Diuretics, such as furosemide (Lasix®) may be used for congestive heart failure.
- ACE inhibitor (Captopril®) to decrease pulmonary hypertension.
- Surgical repair includes pulmonary banding or cardiopulmonary bypass repair of the opening with suturing or a patch, depending upon the size.

Patent Ductus Arteriosus

Patent ductus arteriosus (PDA) is failure of the ductus arteriosus that connects the pulmonary artery and aorta to close after birth, resulting in left to right shunting of blood from the aorta back to the pulmonary artery. This increases the blood flow to the lungs and causes an increase in pulmonary hypertension that can result in damage to the lung tissue. **Symptoms** include:

- Essentially asymptomatic (some infants).
- Cyanosis.
- Congestive heart failure.

95

- Machinery-like murmur.
- Frequent respiratory infections and dyspnea, especially on exertion.
- Widened pulse pressure.
- Bounding pulse.
- Atrial fibrillation/ palpitations.
- Increased risk for bacterial endocarditis, congestive heart failure, and development of pulmonary vascular obstructive disease.

Treatment includes:

- Indomethacin (Indocin®) given within 10 days of birth is successful in closing about 80% of defects.
- Surgical repair with ligation of the patent vessel.

Coarctation of the Aorta

Coarctation of the aorta is a stricture of the aorta, proximal to the ductus arteriosus intersection. The increased blood pressure caused by the heart attempting to pump the blood past the stricture causes the heart to enlarge and also increases blood pressure to the head and upper extremities while decreasing blood pressure to the lower body and extremities. With severe stricture, symptoms may not occur until the ductus arteriosus closes, causing sudden loss of blood supply to the lower body. **Symptoms** include:

- Difference in blood pressure between upper and lower extremities
- Congestive heart failure symptoms in infants.
- Headaches, dizziness, and nosebleeds in older children
- Increased risk of hypertension, ruptured aorta, aortic aneurysm, bacterial endocarditis, and brain attack.

Treatment includes:

- Prostaglandin (alprostadil), such as Prostin VR Pediatric®, to reopen the ductus arteriosus for infants
- Balloon angioplasty
- Surgical resection and anastomosis or graft replacement (usually at 3-5 years of age unless condition is severe). Infants who have surgery may need later repair.

TOF

Tetralogy of Fallot (TOF) is a combination of 4 different defects:

- Ventricular septal defect (usually with a large opening).
- Pulmonic stenosis with decreased blood flow to lungs.
- Overriding aorta (displacement to the right so that it appears to come from both ventricles, usually overriding the ventricular septal defect), resulting in mixing of oxygenated and deoxygenated blood.
- Right ventricular hypertrophy.

Infants are often acutely cyanotic immediately after birth while others with less severe defects may have increasing cyanosis over the first year. **Symptoms** include:

- Intolerance to feeding or crying, resulting in increased cyanotic "blue spells" or "tet spells."
- Failure to thrive with poor growth.
- Clubbing of fingers may occur over time.
- Intolerance to activity as child grows.
- Increased risk for emboli, brain attacks, brain abscess, seizures, fainting or sudden death.

Treatment includes:

- Total surgical repair at 1 year or younger is now the preferred treatment rather than palliative procedures formerly used.

Aortic Stenosis

Aortic stenosis is a stricture (narrowing) of the aortic valve that controls the flow of blood from the left ventricle, causing the left ventricular wall to thicken as it increases pressure to overcome the valvular resistance, increasing afterload, and increasing the need for blood supply from the coronary arteries. This condition may result from a birth defect or childhood rheumatic fever and tends to worsen as over the years as the heart grows. **Symptoms** include:

- Chest pain on exertion and intolerance of exercise
- Heart murmur
- Hypotension on exertion may be associated with sudden fainting.
- Sudden death can occur.
- Tachycardia with faint pulse
- Poor feeding
- Increased risk for bacterial endocarditis and coronary insufficiency.
- Increases mitral regurgitation and secondary pulmonary hypertension.

Treatment in children may be done before symptoms develop because of the danger of sudden death. Treatment includes:

- Balloon valvuloplasty to dilate valve non-surgically.
- Surgical repair of valve or replacement of valve, depending upon the extent of stricture.

Pulmonic Stenosis

Pulmonic stenosis is a stricture of the pulmonic valve that controls the flow of blood from the right ventricle to the lungs, resulting in right ventricular hypertrophy as the pressure increases in the right ventricle and decreased pulmonary blood flow. The condition may be asymptomatic or symptoms may not be evident until the child enters adulthood, depending upon the severity of the defect. Pulmonic stenosis may be associated with a number of other heart defects. **Symptoms** of pulmonic stenosis can include:

- Loud heart murmur
- Congestive heart murmur
- Mild cyanosis
- Cardiomegaly
- Angina

- Dyspnea
- Fainting
- Increased risk of bacterial endocarditis

Treatment includes:

- Balloon valvuloplasty to separate the cusps of the valve for children.
- Surgical repair includes the (closed) transventricular valvotomy (Brock) procedure for infants and the cardiopulmonary bypass pulmonary valvotomy for older children.

HLHS

Hypoplastic left heart syndrome (HLHS) is underdevelopment of the left ventricle and ascending aortic atresia causing inability of the heart to pump blood, so most blood flows from the left atrium through the foramen ovale to the right atrium and to the lungs with the descending aorta receiving blood through the ductus arteriosus. There may be valvular abnormalities as well. Symptoms may be mild until the ductus arteriosus closes at about 2 weeks causing a marked increase in cyanosis and decreased cardiac output. **Symptoms** include:

- Increasing cyanosis.
- Decreased cardiac output leading to cardiovascular collapse.

Mortality rates are 100% without surgical correction and 25% with correction. **Surgical procedures** include a series of 3 staged operations:

- Norwood procedure connects the main pulmonary artery to the aorta, a shunt for pulmonary blood flow, and creates a large atrial septal defect.
- Glenn procedure.
- Fontan repair procedure.
- Heart transplantation in infancy is preferred in many cases, but the shortage of hearts limits this option.

Tricuspid Atresia

Tricuspid atresia is lack of tricuspid valve between the right atrium and right ventricle so blood flows through the foramen ovale or an atrial defect to the left atrium and then through a ventricular wall defect from the left ventricle to the right ventricle and out to the lungs, causing oxygenated and deoxygenated bloods to mix. Pulmonic obstruction is common. **Symptoms** include:

- Cyanosis obvious postnatally.
- Tachycardia and dyspnea.
- Increasing hypoxemia and clubbing in older children.
- Increased risk for bacterial endocarditis, brain abscess, and brain attack.

Treatment includes:

- Prostaglandin (alprostadil), to keep the ductus arteriosus and foramen ovale open if there are no septal defects.
- Numerous surgical procedures, including pulmonary artery banding, shunting from the aorta to the pulmonary arteries, Glenn procedure (connecting superior vena cava to pulmonary artery to allow deoxygenated blood to flow to the lungs), atrial septostomy to enlarge the opening between the atria, and the Fontan corrective procedure (usually done at 2-4 years after previous stabilizing procedures).

Transposition of Great Arteries

Transposition of great arteries is the aorta and pulmonary artery arising from the wrong ventricle (aorta from the right ventricle and pulmonary artery from the left), so there is no connection between pulmonary and systemic circulation with deoxygenated blood being pumped back to the body and the oxygenated blood from the lungs is pumped back to the lungs. Septal defects may also occur, allowing some mixing of blood and the ductus arteriosus allows mixing until it closes. **Symptoms** vary depending upon whether there is mixing of blood but may include:

- Mild to severe cyanosis
- Symptoms of congestive heart failure
- Cardiomegaly develops in the weeks after birth.
- Heart sounds vary depending upon the severity of the defects.

Treatment may include:

- Prostaglandin to keep the ductus arteriosus and foramen ovale open. Balloon atrial septostomy to increase size of foramen ovale.
- Surgical repair to transpose arteries to the normal position ("arterial switch") as well of repair septal defects and other abnormalities.

Total Anomalous Pulmonary Venous Return

Total anomalous pulmonary venous return is a defect in which the 4 pulmonary veins connect to the right atrium by an anomalous connection rather than the right atrium so there is no direct blood flow to the left side of the heart; however, an atrial septal defect is common and allows for the mixed oxygenated and deoxygenated blood to shunt to the left and enter the aorta. There are 4 different types of anomalies, and in some cases pulmonary vein obstruction. If the pulmonary veins are not obstructed, children may be asymptomatic initially. **Symptoms** include:

- Heart murmur.
- Severe post-natal cyanosis or mild cyanosis.
- Dyspnea with grunting and sternal retraction or dyspnea on exertion
- Low oxygen saturation (in the 80s if there is no pulmonary obstruction).
- Cardiomegaly (right-sided hypertrophy)

Treatment includes:

- Surgical repair to attach the pulmonary veins to the left atrium and correct any other defects may be done immediately after birth or delayed for 1-2 months.

Truncus Arteriosus

Truncus arteriosus is the blood from both ventricles flowing into one large artery with one valve, with more blood flowing to the lower pressure pulmonary arteries than to the body, resulting in low oxygen saturation and hypoxemia. Usually, there is a ventricular septal defect so the blood mixes across the ventricles. **Symptoms** include:

- Congestive heart failure with pulmonary edema because of increased blood flow to lungs.
- Typical symptoms of congestive heart failure.
- Cyanosis, especially about the face (mouth and nose).
- Dyspnea, increasing on feeding or exertion.
- Poor feeding and failure to thrive.
- Heart murmur.
- Increased risk for brain abscess and bacterial endocarditis.

Treatment includes:

- Palliative banding of the pulmonary arteries to decrease the flow of blood to the lungs.
- Surgical repair with cardiopulmonary bypass includes closing the ventricular defect, utilizing the existing single artery as the aorta by separating the pulmonary arteries from it and creating a conduit between the pulmonary arteries and the right ventricle.

Cardiac Dysrhythmias

Cardiac dysrhythmias, abnormal heart beats, are more common in adults can occur and are frequently the result of damage to the conduction system during major cardiac surgery.

Bradydysrhythmia are pulse rates that are abnormally slow:

- *Complete atrioventricular block (A-V block)* may be congenital or a response to surgical trauma.
- *Sinus bradycardia* may be caused by the autonomic nervous system or a response to hypotension and decrease in oxygenation.
- *Junctional/nodal rhythms* often occur in post-surgical patients when absence of P wave is noted but heart rate and output usually remain stable, and unless there is compromise, usually no treatment is necessary.

Tachydysrhythmia are pulse rates that are abnormally fast:

- *Sinus tachycardia* is often caused by illness, such as fever or infection.
- *Supraventricular tachycardia* (200-300 bpm) may have a sudden onset and result in congestive heart failure.

Conduction irregularities are irregular pulses that often occur post-operatively and are usually not significant:

- *Premature contractions* may arise from the atria or ventricles.

Complete A-V Block

Complete atrioventricular block (A-V block) may be congenital or acquired as a response to surgical trauma and has become more common in infants and children as survival rates for cardiac surgery improve. It is categorized as 3rd degree AV block, in which there are more P waves than QRS and there is no clear relationship between them. The atrial rate may be 2-3 times the pulse rate. If the SA node malfunctions, the AV node can fire at a lower rate, and if the AV node malfunctions, there is a pacemaker site in the ventricles that will take over at a bradycardic rate; thus, even with complete AV block, the heart still contracts, but often very ineffectually. The heart may be able to compensate at rest, but can't keep pace with exertion. The resultant bradycardia may cause congestive heart failure, fainting, or even sudden death, and usually conduction abnormalities slowly worsen. All patients with complete AV block are normally treated with implanted pacemakers, usually dual chamber pacemakers.

Use of Pacemakers in Children

Children receive **pacemakers** primarily for third-degree atrioventricular block, sinus bradycardia, and atrioventricular block that occurs after surgery. Some heart transplant patients may require pacemakers. The parts of the pacemaker include one or two pacing leads (which may elude steroids) that attach to the atrial or ventricular myocardium, or the epicardium in some cases, to sense electrical impulses, leading to an implantable pulse generator (IPG) that contains a lithium battery and microprocessors. In small children, the pacemakers may be placed in the abdomen rather than the shoulder area, which is used for older children. The choice of single or double lead pacemakers depends upon the condition of the heart and whether the arrhythmias are atrial, ventricular, or both. The pacemaker is set for the individual and detects electrical impulses and delivers an impulse if it is missing and can be reset non-invasively. Pacemakers prevent the pulse from falling below a certain rate, but also can adjust for activity.

Use of ICDs in Children

The **implantable cardioverter defibrillator (ICD)** is similar to the pacemaker and is implanted in the same way with one or more leads to the ventricular myocardium or the epicardium, but it is used to control tachycardia or fibrillation. Severe tachycardia may be related to electrical disturbances, cardiomyopathy, or postoperative response to repair of congenital disease. In some cases, it is not responsive to medications. When the pulse reaches a certain preset rate, then the device automatically provides a small electrical impulse to the atrial or ventricular myocardium to slow the heart. If fibrillation occurs, a higher energy shock is delivered. It takes 5-15 seconds for the device to detect abnormalities in the pulse rate and more than one shock may be required, so fainting can occur. Some devices can function as both a pacemaker and an ICD, especially important for children who have both episodes of bradycardia and tachycardia.

Hypertensive Crises

Hypertensive crises in children are usually related to acute glomerulonephritis, renal hypertension, drug abuse, intracranial hemorrhage, and perioperative hypertension. Hypertensive crises are classified according to severity:

- *Hypertensive emergency* occurs when acute hypertension (1.5 x the 95th percentile) must be treated immediately to lower blood pressure in order to prevent damage to vital organs, such as left ventricular hypertrophy or retinopathy. It is usually associated with dissecting aortic aneurysm, myocardial infarction, and intracranial hemorrhage. Medications that act very quickly are usually administered: vasodilators such as nitroprusside (Nipride®, Nitropress®) and nitroglycerine.

- *Hypertensive urgency* occurs when acute hypertension must be treated within a few hours but the vital organs are not in immediate danger. This is the most common type for children. Blood pressure is lowered more slowly to avoid hypotension, ischemia of vital organs, or failure of autoregulation. Usually lowering occurs by the following:
    - 1/3 reduction in 6 hours
    - 1/3 reduction in next 24 hours
    - 1/3 reduction over days 2-4

Mitral Valve

The **mitral valve** (left atrioventricular valve) is located between the left atrium and the left ventricle. It is a bicuspid valve in that is comprised of two leaflets, which are circled by a fibrotic ring called the mitral valve annulus. The chordae tendineae are tendons attached to the posterior surface (ventricular side) of the leaflets on one end and the finger-like projecting papillary muscles of the ventricle wall on the other, preventing prolapse of the valve back into the atrium. When the left ventricle contracts, the chordae tendineae essentially pulls and holds the valve closed. When ventricular pressure relaxes (during left ventricular diastole), the mitral valve opens and blood (80%) from the left atrium flows through into the left ventricle. Then, the left atrium contracts, sending more blood (20%) through the valve. As the left ventricle begins to contract, the valve closes and blood flows from the left ventricle to the aorta and the systemic circulation.

Mitral Stenosis and Pulmonary Hypertension

Mitral stenosis is caused by an autoimmune response to rheumatic fever leading to vegetative growths on the mitral valve. It can also be caused by infective endocarditis or lupus erythematosus. Over time, the leaflets thicken and calcify and the commissures (junctions) fuse, decreasing the size of the valve opening. Mitral stenosis reduces the flow of blood from the left atrium to the left ventricle. Pressure in the left atrium increases to overcome resistance, resulting in enlargement of the left atrium and increased pressure in the pulmonary veins and capillaries of the lung. *Symptoms of exertional dyspnea usually occur when the valve is 50% occluded.* There are 3 mechanisms by which mitral stenosis causes pulmonary hypertension.

- Increased left atrial pressure causing backward increase in pressure of pulmonary veins.
- Hypertrophy and pulmonary artery constriction resulting from reactive left atrial and pulmonary venous hypertension.
- Thrombotic/embolic damage to pulmonary vasculature.

Treatment includes drugs to control arrhythmias and hypertension, balloon valvuloplasty, and mitral valve replacement.

Mitral Valve Regurgitation

Mitral valve regurgitation may occur with mitral stenosis or independently. It can result from damage caused by rheumatic fever, myxomatous degeneration caused by a genetic defect in the valvular collagen, infective endocarditis, collagen vascular disease (Marfan's syndrome) or cardiomyopathy. Hypertrophy and dilation of the left ventricle may cause displacement of the leaflets and dilation of the valve. Regurgitation occurs when the mitral valve fails to close completely so that there is backflow into the left atrium from the left ventricle during systole, decreasing cardiac output. There are 3 phases:

- *Acute* may occur with rupture of a chordae tendineae or papillary muscle causing sudden left ventricular flooding and overload.
- *Chronic compensated* results in enlargement of the left atrium to decrease filling pressure and hypertrophy of the left ventricle to maintain stroke volume and cardiac output.
- *Chronic decompensated* occurs when the left ventricle fails to compensate for the volume overload so that stroke volume and cardiac output decrease.

Review of Systems: Renal

Renal Anatomy and Physiology

Renal Pelvis and Glomerulus

The kidneys are a pair of organs located behind the peritoneal cavity on the posterior wall of the abdomen. In children, they are larger, proportionately, than they are in adults. There are 2 regions to the kidney:

- *Renal pelvis (hilum):* The concave area through which the renal artery and vein enter and exit, and from which urine drains into the ureter. The renal artery, from the abdominal aorta, divides into smaller arterioles and eventually becomes the glomerulus (capillary bed responsible for glomerular filtration) in the cortex. *The glomerulus* has 3 filtering layers: the capillary endothelium, the basement membrane, and the epithelium, which filters blood and removes fluid and small molecules but prevents passage of blood cells, albumin, and larger molecules. Blood returns from the glomerulus through the renal pelvis to the inferior vena cava.

Renal Parenchyma

Renal parenchyma is divided two parts:

- *Renal cortex:* Outer portion of the kidney beneath the capsule, containing nephrons. *The nephron* is the functional unit of the cortex with about 1 million nephrons per kidney. The nephron comprises:
  - Glomerulus with afferent and efferent arterials.
  - Bowman's capsule
  - Proximal tubule
  - Loop of Henle
  - Distal tubule
  - Collecting ducts, which converge into papillae.

Urine forms in the nephrons through a 3-step process:

- *Glomerular filtration:* filters water, electrolytes, glucose, urea, and creatinine from blood entering from the afferent arteriole.
- *Tubular reabsorption:* Some of the filtered substances are reabsorbed through the peritubular capillaries to the renal vein.
- *Tubular secretion:* Remainder is excreted in urine.

- *Renal medulla*: 8-18 fan-shaped renal pyramids, with each forming a lobe with the adjacent cortex. The tips of the renal pyramids (papillae), empty into 4-13 minor calices, to 2-3 major calices, and from there to the renal pelvis.

Bladder Exstrophy

Bladder exstrophy is eversion of posterior wall of the bladder through the anterior wall of the bladder and through the lower abdominal wall with bladder and urethra exposed, a wide pubic arch, anterior displacement of the anus, renal disorders, and abnormalities of reproductive organs in both males and females. Symptoms include urinary and bowel problems related to specific anomalies. Diagnosis is by physical examination to assess abnormalities. Renal ultrasound is done to determine the number of kidneys and presence of hydroureteronephrosis.

Treatment is as follows:

First stage:

- Primary closure of bladder: No ostomy necessary if done within 72 hours of birth. Procedures include ureteral stents and suprapubic urinary drainage.
- Bilateral iliac ostomies: Necessary after 72 hours because pelvic ring is not malleable.
- Epispadias repair: May be done in first or second stage.

Second stage:

- Epispadias repair: Usually done between 6-12 months.

Final stage:

- Bladder neck reconstruction and reimplantation of ureters.
- Permanent urinary diversion: Required by 10-15%.

Posterior Urethral Valves

Posterior urethral valves are a urethral abnormality in males where urethral valves have narrow slit-like openings that impede flow and allow reverse flow, damaging urinary organs, which swell and become engorged with urine. 30% will develop long-term kidney failure. **Symptoms** vary, depending upon severity:

- Dysuria: Pain, weak stream, frequency. Hematuria. Urinary retention. Incontinence. Enlarged bladder palpable as abdominal mass. Urinary infection (most common after 1 year of age). Sepsis, metabolic acidosis, and azotemia (increased blood levels of urea and other nitrogenous compounds) may develop.

Diagnosis includes the following:

Fetal ultrasound
- *Voiding cystourethrogram (VCUG):* Evaluate extent of valvular abnormality and other urinary defects.
- *Endoscopy:* Examine inside of urinary tract/take tissue samples. *Blood tests:* Assess kidney function and electrolytes.

104

Treatment includes the following:

- *Medical management:* Supportive care, antibiotics, electrolytes, Foley catheter.
- *Urinary diversion:* Usually closed after valve repair.
- *Endoscopic ablation/resection:* Examine obstruction and remove valve leaflets.

Enuresis

Enuresis is repeated involuntary urinary incontinence in children old enough to have bladder control, usually about 5-6 years old. Diabetes and other disorders should be ruled out although 95% are not associated with structural or neurological disorders. There are **3 types**:

- *Primary:* The child has never been dry at night, and incontinence is associated with delay in maturation and small functional bladder rather than stress or psychiatric disorders.
- *Intermittent:* The child stays dry part of the time with episodes of incontinence at night.
- *Secondary:* The child has had long periods (6-12 months) staying dry and then is incontinent because of infection, stress, or sleep disorder.

Treatment includes:

- Laboratory assessment and examination to rule out primary causes.
- Fluid restriction.
- Bladder training and enuresis alarms.
- Imipramine (tricyclic antidepressant) is used with many children but require close monitoring.
- Desmopressin nasal spray may be used for short-term control.
- Support and acceptance.

Prune Belly (Eagle-Barrett) Syndrome

Prune belly (Eagle-Barrett) syndrome is a group of abnormalities involving lack of developed abdominal muscles, undescended testicles, and urinary tract problems. Urinary abnormalities may include large, hypotonic bladder, dilated ureters, and prostatic urethra. Males comprise 96-99% of cases. It may include anomalies of the pulmonary, cardiac, skeletal, and GI tracts. **Symptoms** vary widely, frequently including cardio-pulmonary complications:

- *Prune-like appearance of abdomen*: from fetal abdominal distention. After birth, abdominal fluid is lost and abdomen develops wrinkled "prune" appearance, noticeable because of undeveloped abdominal muscles.
- Undescended testicles: Bilaterally.
- *Urinary tract abnormalities:* Urinary infections, obstruction, and chronic renal failure.

Diagnosis is by physical examination; chest x-rays to evaluate pulmonary problems, renal ultrasound to evaluate kidneys, and voiding cystourethrogram (VCUG) to evaluate urinary defects.

Treatment: Monitor condition. Antibiotics, therapeutic and prophylactic. Intermittent catheterization.

Surgical repair to correct genitourinary defects varies according to abnormality. Procedures may include:

- Vesicostomy, ureterostomy, or pyelostomy. Reduction cystoplasty, urethroplasty. Abdominoplasty

Megaureter

Megaureter is dilation of ureters from the normal 3-5mm to more than 10mm in diameter with or without obstruction and/or reflux from abnormality of ureters or secondary causes:

- *Primary obstruction:* At point where ureter joins bladder; can cause kidney damage. *Refluxing:* Backward flow of urine from bladder to ureters. *Non-obstructing/non-refluxing:* Dilated ureters without blockage may resolve over time. *Obstructed/ refluxing:* Ureters continue to dilate with blockage.
- *Secondary:* Ureters enlarge because of other conditions, such as neurogenic bladder.

Symptoms include urinary tract infection, dysuria, back/flank pain, and fever.

Diagnosis is by:

- *Fetal ultrasound: in utero* diagnosis. *Ultrasound:* To evaluate appearance of urinary tract. *Voiding cystourethrogram (VCUG):* To check for reflux.
- *Diuretic renal scan:* To check for obstruction.
- *Intravenous pyelogram:* To view urinary system.

Treatment includes the following:

- Antibiotic prophylaxis: Until surgery.
- *Ureteral implantation*: Trimming widened portion of ureter; removing obstruction and reattaching.

Ureteropelvic Junction Obstruction

Ureteropelvic junction obstruction (UPI) is congenital obstruction at point where ureter connects to renal pelvis, unilaterally or bilaterally, causing inadequate urinary flow and hydronephrosis. Some children improve markedly within first 18 months, but others require surgery. **Symptoms** include:

- Urinary tract infections. Abdominal or flank pain
- Palpable mass from hydronephrosis. Vomiting.

Diagnosis is based on:

- Fetal ultrasound: in utero diagnosis.
- *Renal ultrasound:* To show dilation of renal pelvis.
- Intravenous pyelogram (IVP): To identify obstruction.
- *Renal isotope scan:* To evaluate and measure kidney function.

Treatment includes the following:

- Fetal urinary diversion: Remains controversial.
- *Pyeloplasty:* Open surgical procedure where ureteropelvic junction is excised and ureter reattached to renal pelvis with wide junction, allowing adequate drainage.
- *Laparoscopic pyeloplasty:* Through abdominal wall and abdominal cavity with internal excision of ureteropelvic junction.
- *Insertion of wire through ureter:* To cut ureteropelvic junction from inside with a ureteral drain left in place for a few weeks.

Neurogenic Bladder

Neurogenic bladder is bladder dysfunction from lesions of peripheral or central nervous system, related to traumatic or congenital etiologies or develop from cerebrovascular accident or diabetic neuropathy. Nerve damage can cause under-active bladder unable to contract to effectively empty the bladder or overactive bladder that contracts frequently and ineffectually. **Symptoms** vary:

- *Under-active:* Incontinence, dribbling, straining or inability to urinate, retention.
- *Overactive:* Frequency, urgency, dysuria, urinary tract infection, fever.

Diagnosis is by:

Neurological testing (x-rays, MRI, and EEGs): To determine etiology. *24-hour urine collection:* To determine volume and urine patterns. *Bladder stress test:* To determine reaction to full bladder while bending over, coughing, walking, or doing other activities.

Treatment includes the following:

- *Antibiotics:* To control infections.
- Clean intermittent catheterization (CIC): To empty bladder.
- *Endoscopy:* Combined with cutting of external sphincter or injecting sphincter with paralytic agents to allow urination.
- *Surgical repair:* Placing of permanent stents at bladder neck, bladder augmentation to increase bladder size, repair of vesicoureteral reflux, or urinary diversion.

Vesicoureteral Reflux

Vesicoureteral reflux is an abnormality where urine flows from bladder back up ureters. Reflux is graded on international scale of 1-5, depending upon degree of dilation of ureter and renal pelvis.

- *Primary:* Congenital defect with impaired valve where ureter opens to bladder. The ureter may be too short so the valve doesn't close properly. *Secondary:* Caused by infection or other cause of obstruction.

Symptoms of urinary tract infection are most common:

- *Neonates:* Fever, irritability, lethargy, emesis.
- *Older infants, children:* Abdominal pain, emesis, diarrhea, fever, dysuria with enuresis, frequency, urgency, cloudy/foul urine. *Late symptoms:* Hypertension, dysuria with difficulty urinating, proteinuria, chronic renal insufficiency.

Diagnosis is by:

- *Ultrasound:* Evaluate appearance of urinary system.
- *Voiding cystourethrogram (VCUG):* Identify reflux (after infection has cleared). *Intravenous pyelogram:* Reveal obstructions. *Nuclear scans:* Show urinary functioning
- *Cystoscopy:* View bladder interior.

Treatment includes the following:

- *Antibiotics*: For infection.
- *Surgical repair/reconstruction:* Usually involves severing ureter from bladder and reattaching at a different angle to prevent reflux.

Chronic Renal Failure

Renal failure occurs when the kidneys are unable to filter and excrete wastes, concentrate urine, and maintain electrolyte balance because of hypoxic conditions, kidney disease, or obstruction in the urinary tract. It results first in azotemia (increase in nitrogenous waste in the blood) and then in uremia (nitrogenous wastes cause toxic symptoms.) When >50% of the functional renal capacity is destroyed, the kidneys can no longer carry out necessary functions and progressive deterioration begins over months or years. Symptoms are often non-specific in the beginning with loss of appetite and energy. **Symptoms** and complications include:

- Weight loss. Headaches, muscle cramping, general malaise. ↑Bruising and dry or itching skin.
- ↑ BUN and creatinine.
- Sodium and fluid retention with edema.
- Hyperkalemia. Metabolic acidosis.
- Calcium and phosphorus depletion, resulting in altered bone metabolism, pain, and retarded growth.
- Anemia with decreased production on RBCs.
- Increased risk of infection. Uremic syndrome.

Treatment includes the following:

- Supportive/symptomatic therapy.
- Dialysis and transplantation.

Persistent Cloaca

Persistent cloaca is a condition in females with an imperforate anus and the rectum, vagina, and urethra forming a single channel with a rectal fistula attached to the posterior wall of the channel. **Diagnosis** is made with a physical exam showing a single perineal opening. An abdominal mass (hydrocolpos—distended bladder) may occur. A voiding cystourethrogram (VCUG) will show bladder abnormalities if catheterization is possible.

Treatment includes the following:

- *Colostomy:* Fecal diversion in neonate prevents fecal material from entering urinary system and causing infection.
- *Decompression of vagina:* Prevents infection and scarring and relieves obstruction of urinary tract.

- *Posterior Sagittal Anorectovagino-Urethroplasty* (PSARVUP): (Usually 2 months after colostomy.) Rectum is separated from vagina, vagina is separated from urethra, urethra is reconstructed, vagina is reconstructed, and rectum is reconstructed with anoplasty,
- *Postoperative anal dilation:* 2 weeks after surgery until final size is reached.
- *Cystoscopy/ Vaginoscopy:* Checks for urethrovaginal fistula.
- *Colostomy removal:* Anastomosis of colon and rectum and colostomy removed.

Obstructive Uropathy Resulting in Hydronephrosis

Hydronephrosis is collection of urine in the renal pelvis causing cyst-like distention and compression damage of renal parenchyma above an area of obstruction. It occurs more frequently in boys and is often associated with other abnormalities (prune belly syndrome, hypospadias, and genetic abnormalities). Chronic obstructive uropathy can damage distal nephrons, interfering with ability to concentrate urine, increasing urine flow, and causing metabolic acidosis. The pooled urine increases urinary infections. Partial obstruction causes progressive loss of function. Hydronephrosis may be **caused** by a number of different conditions:

- Bladder outlet obstruction in the urethra or bladder opening may occur in both male and female newborns. Male newborns may exhibit posterior urethral valves (slit-like opening in the urethra that creates backflow of urine).
- Ureterocele causing obstruction.
- Ureteropelvic junction obstruction, usually only in one kidney.
- Vesicoureteral reflex prevents urine from completely entering bladder so there is reflux up the ureter to the kidney.

Polycystic Kidney Disease

Polycystic kidney disease (PK) is caused by renal cysts (fluid-filled sacs in renal tissue), which may be genetic or acquired. The cysts develop from nephrons and can cause gross enlargement of kidneys. Cysts may be single or multiple (polycystic) and may involve one or both kidneys. PK is often associated with cystic disease in other organs as well. There are 3 **types** of PK:

- *Autosomal dominant* is the most common (90%), but symptoms are usually delayed until adulthood although they can occur in childhood. However, it may progress to ESRD over time. *Symptoms* include urinary and cyst infections, rupture of cysts with hematuria, hypertension and renal calculi.
- *Autosomal recessive* is rarer and symptoms arise much earlier, sometimes in the fetus.
- *Acquired* usually does not affect children because it develops from long-term kidney disease or dialysis.

Treatment cannot cure but can delay effects:

- Antihypertensives.
- Antibiotics for infections.
- Analgesia.
- Growth hormone (autosomal recessive).
- Long-term: dialysis and transplantation.

Hemolytic Uremic Syndrome

Hemolytic uremic syndrome is a life-threatening disorder usually follows an *E. coli* infection. Mortality rates are 3-5%, but chronic renal problems develop in 50% and a few have lifelong complications, including blindness, paralysis, and kidney failure requiring dialysis. **Symptoms** include:

- Weakness, lethargy.
- Nausea and increased diarrhea.
- Fever.
- Hematuria and decreased urinary output.
- Petechiae and ecchymosis.
- Blood in the stool.
- Jaundice.
- Alterations in consciousness.
- Seizures (rare).
- Bleeding from the nose or mouth.
- Hypertension.
- Edema.
- Paralysis (cerebral blood clot).

Treatment includes:

- Antibiotics are contraindicated unless sepsis is present.
- Intravenous fluids and nutritional supplements.
- Blood transfusions may be needed.
- Plasmapheresis is sometimes used to remove antibodies from the blood.
- Protein limitation and ACE inhibitors to prevent permanent kidney damage.

Obstructive Uropathy with Nephrosis

Obstructive uropathy with nephrosis may present with a variety of **symptoms** depending upon the underlying cause, but most include:

- Pain in flank area.
- Recurrent urinary infections with associated pain and fever.
- Dysuria decreased urinary output, foul urine, and/or hematuria.
- Edema.
- Renal failure.

Sometimes obstructions will resolve over time and may not constitute medical emergencies, especially if only one side is involved. However, if blockage is causing severe symptoms or does not resolve, various **treatments** may be used:

- Prenatal shunts may be done if the condition is identified through ultrasound although the procedure carries risk so it is done primarily if the life of the fetus is threatened,
- Ureteral/urethral stent may be inserted to maintain patency of ureter.
- Urinary diversions, such as ileal conduit or cutaneous ureterostomy may be indicated in cases of severe obstruction, especially those associated with congenital abnormalities.
- Antibiotics for infections.

Fluid Balance in Infants and Children

Body fluid is primarily intracellular fluid (ICF) or extracellular space (ECF). Infants and children have proportionately more extracellular fluid (ECF) than adults. At birth, more than half of the child's weight is ECF, but by 3 years of age, the balance is more like adults:

- ECF: 20-30% (interstitial fluid, plasma, transcellular fluid).
- ICF: 40-50% (fluid within the cells).

The fluid compartments are separated by semipermeable membranes that allow fluid and solutes (electrolytes and other substances) to move by osmosis. Fluid also moves through diffusion, filtration, and active transport. In fluid volume deficit, fluid is out of balance and ECF is depleted; an overload occurs with increased concentration of sodium and retention of fluid. Signs of **fluid deficit** include:

- Thirsty, restless to lethargic.
- Increasing pulse rate, tachycardia.
- Fontanels depressed (infants).
- ↓ Urinary output.
- Normal BP progressing to hypotension.
- Dry mucous membranes.
- 3-10% ↓ in body weight.

Review of Systems: Reproductive

Phimosis and Cryptorchidism

Phimosis is narrowing or stenosis of the foreskin. If the condition is mild, retracting the foreskin may dilate it sufficiently, but in more severe cases, circumcision or vertical incision and suturing may be necessary. About 12% of males not circumcised at birth will develop phimosis, sometimes as the result of infection. Betamethasone cream 0.5% applied twice daily for a month to the glans penis may be effective and avoid surgery.

Cryptorchidism, failure of one or both testicles to descend through the inguinal canal into the scrotum, occurs in 30% of premature males and 3-4% of full-term male infants. Cryptorchidism may result from deficiency of testosterone, structural abnormalities, or absent or defective testis. In 75%, the condition resolves ≤3 months. If it persists, human chorionic gonadotropin may be given to detect non-palpable testis, and then surgical repair is done at 1 year to prevent damage to the testicle. If the testis is defective, it is surgically removed to reduce incidence of cancer.

Epispadias and Hypospadias

Epispadias is the urethral orifice in an abnormal position with a widened pubic bone. In boys, the urethra may open on the top (dorsum), the sides, or the complete length of the penis; in girls, the urethra, with a urethral cleft along its length, usually bifurcates the clitoris and labia but may be in the abdomen. Boys may have a short, wide penis with abnormal chordee (curvature). It is 3-5 times more common in males than females.

Hypospadias is the urethral orifice opening onto the ventral surface of the penis. Diagnosis is by physical exam and endoscopy to evaluate bladder neck and external sphincter. Intravenous pyelogram evaluates the urinary tract. Symptoms include urinary incontinence, infections, reflux nephropathy (backward flow of urine to kidneys).

Surgical repair may include lengthening of the urethra and penis in males as well as bladder neck reconstruction. May require multiple surgical procedures to complete reconstruction for both males and females. Urinary diversion may be necessary if incontinence cannot be corrected.

Adolescent Menstrual Disorders

Menarche occurs between 9-15 in most girls, preceded by development of secondary sexual characteristics. The usual menstrual cycle is every 21-35 days, lasting 2-7 days with blood loss of 35-150 mL/monthly cycle. **Menstrual disorders** may cause considerable discomfort:

- *Dysmenorrhea* is pain associated with menses, usually 6-24 months after menarche. Pain usually lasts about 2 days and is accompanied by mild to severe cramping in the supra-pubic area, lumbar back, and labia. **Treatment** includes:
    - NSAIDs (Ibuprofen 400-900mg/4 times daily
    - Naproxen 250-500 mg every 6-12 hours.)
- *Endometriosis* occurs when endometrial tissue outside of the pelvic area irritates nerve endings and causes severe pain and uterine cramping during periods, usually preceded by a few days of increasing dysmenorrhea. **Treatment** consists of the following:
    - Referral to gynecologist
    - NSAIDs
    - Oral contraceptives to reduce shedding
    - Gonadotropin-releasing hormone to reduce estrogen and androgen levels
    - laparoscopy to remove extrauterine endometrial tissue.
- *Dysfunctional uterine bleeding* results from an abnormality in hormones so that shedding of the endometrium is irregular, resulting in excessive bleeding or irregular periods. **Treatment** includes:
    - Hgb >12: NSAIDs with iron supplementation.
    - Hgb 10-12 add folic acid supplement.
    - Hgb <10 may require hospitalization or referral to gynecologist.
- *Mittelschmerz* is pain in the middle of the menstrual cycle, usually dull in the lower abdomen and lasting for minutes to hours, and probably related to enlargement of follicle before rupture. **Treatment** includes the following:
    - Heating pad may relieve discomfort.
    - NSAIDs.
- *Amenorrhea* may be primary (absence ≤16 years) with normal pubertal development (within 3 years) or with no pubertal development. It may also be secondary (no periods for 3 cycles/6 months), related to excessive exercise or dieting. Primary and secondary amenorrhea requires testing to determine if there are abnormalities in hormones, genetic disorders, obstructive disorders, or other causes. **Treatment** depends on underlying cause.

Review of Systems: Neurological

Manifestations of Spinal Cord Injury

Spinal cord injury is less common in young children than adults with the highest incidence between ages 16-30, primarily occurring as the result of automobile or sporting accidents although shooting and knifing assaults are also implicated. Automobile accidents may cause spinal cord injury even without vertebral fracture if children are not properly restrained. The degree of disability relates to the level of injury. The areas most commonly injured are those with the greatest mobility: 5-7th cervical, 12th thoracic and 1st lumbar. Damage may vary:

- *Transient* with contusion and bruising with complete recovery.
- *Laceration/ compression* with some resultant paresis.
- *Transection* with complete paralysis below the area of injury: paraplegia or quadriplegia.

Injuries may be primary with direct trauma to the spinal cord, or secondary resulting from a physiological response to contusion, resulting in ischemia, edema, and hemorrhage that cause destruction of the myelin sheaths and axons. Secondary injuries are often reversible if treated within 4-6 hours.

Central Cord, Anterior Cord, and Lateral Cord Syndromes

Incomplete transection or injury to the **spinal cord** can manifest with different **syndromes**:

- *Central cord syndrome*: Injury to central portion of spinal cord, surrounded by undamaged tissue, usually in the cervical area. Usually there are varying degrees of loss of motor ability and sensation in the upper chest and arms. The trunk area may suffer incomplete loss of sensation and control, and bowel and bladder control may remain intact.
- *Anterior cord syndrome:* Injury to anterior portion of spinal cord, usually as the result of herniated disks, hyperflexion injuries, or damage to the anterior spinal artery. There is loss of pain, thermal sensation, and motor function below the injury, but sensations of touch, position, and vibration are intact.
- *Lateral cord syndrome*: Injury to the right or left half of spinal cord, usually from transverse hemisection by knife injury or fracture dislocations. It is characterized by ipsilateral (same side) paralysis and contralateral (opposite side) loss of pain and thermal sensation below injury.

Treatment for Acute Spinal Cord Injuries

Immediate assessment is critical for acute spinal cord injuries to ensure that **treatment** can prevent damage by secondary injury:

- *Airway support* may include suctioning, insertional of oral airway or endotracheal intubation with mechanical ventilation.
- *Hypotension* support with intravenous fluids and assessment is necessary to determine if the cause is neurogenic shock or occult hemorrhage.
- *Nasogastric tube* is used to prevent ileus and aspiration.
- *Spinal radiography:* CT or MRI is often needed to determine the degree of spinal cord injury.
- *Evaluation* for concomitant head injury: neurological exam and CT may be indicated.
- *Methylprednisolone* (Solu-Medrol®) or *Tirilazad* for 24 hours if started within 3 hours, for 48 hours if started within 3-8 hours may be of benefit (studies are inconclusive).
- *Supplementary oxygen* is given for pulmonary support.
- *Positioning and support* must be done to prevent pressure sores.

Spina Bifida and Myelomeningocele

The terms **spina bifida and myelomeningocele** are often used interchangeably, but there is a distinction. Spina bifida is a neural tube defect with an incomplete spinal cord and often missing vertebrae that allow the meninges and spinal cord to protrude through the opening. There are 5 basic types:

- *Spina bifida:* Defect in which the vertebral column is not closed with varying degrees of herniation through the opening.
- *Spina bifida occulta:* Failure of the vertebral column to close, but no herniation through the opening so the defect may not be obvious.
- Spina bifida cystica: Defect in closure with external sac-like protrusion with varying degrees of nerve involvement.
- *Meningocele*: Spina bifida cystica with meningeal sac filled with spinal fluid.
- *Myelomeningocele*: Spina bifida cystica with meningeal sac containing spinal fluid and part of the spinal cord and nerves.

Physical Manifestations and Management Related to Myelomeningocele

Myelomeningocele, which involves spina bifida cystica with a meningeal sac containing spinal fluid and part of the spinal cord and nerves, comprises about 75% of the total cases of spina bifida. There are numerous physical manifestations.

- *Exposed sac* poses the danger of infection and cerebrospinal fluid leakage; so surgical repair is usually done within the first 48 hours although it may be delayed for a few days, especially if the sac is intact.
- *Chiari type II* malformation comprises hypoplasia of the cerebellum and displacement of the lower brainstem into the upper cervical area, which impairs circulation of spinal fluid. It may result in symptoms of cranial nerve dysfunction (dysphonia, dysphagia) and weakness and lack of coordination of upper extremities.
- *Neurogenic bladder* is common and may require credé massage for infants and later intermittent clean catheterization.
- *Fecal incontinence* is common and may be controlled, as the child gets older with diet and bowel training.
- *Musculoskeletal abnormalities* depend upon the level of the myelomeningocele and the degree of impairment but often involve the muscle and joints of the lower extremities and sometimes the upper. Dysfunction often increases with the number of shunts. Scoliosis and lumbar lordosis are common. Hip contractures may cause dislocations.
- *Paralysis/paresis* may vary considerably and be spastic or flaccid. Many children require wheelchairs for mobility although some are fitted with braces for assisted ambulation.
- *Seizures* occur in about a quarter of those affected, sometimes related to shunt malfunction.
- *Hydrocephalus* is present in about 25-35% of infants at birth and 60-70% after surgical repair with ventriculoperitoneal shunt. Untreated, the ventricles will dilate and brain damage can occur.
- *Tethered spinal cord* occurs when the distal end of the spinal cord becomes attached to the bone or site of surgical repair and does not move superiorly with growth, causing increased pain, spasticity, and disability and requiring surgical repair.

Hydrocephalus

The ventricular system produces and circulates cerebrospinal fluid (CSF). There are right and left lateral ventricles, which open into the third ventricle at the interventricular foramen (foramen of Monro). The aqueduct of Sylvius connects the third and fourth ventricles. The fourth ventricle, anterior to the cerebellum, supplies CSF to the subarachnoid space and the spinal cord (dorsal surface). The CSF circulates and then returns to the brain and is absorbed in the arachnoid villi.

Hydrocephalus occurs when there is an imbalance between production and absorption of cerebrospinal fluid in the ventricles, resulting from impaired absorption or obstruction, which may be congenital or acquired. There are primarily 2 types of hydrocephalus that affect children:

- *Communicating*: CSF flows (communicates) between the ventricles but is not absorbed in the subarachnoid space (arachnoid villi).
- *Noncommunicating*: CSF is obstructed (non-communicating) between the ventricles with obstruction, often stenosis of the aqueduct of Sylvius but it can occur anywhere in the system.

Symptoms

Symptoms of hydrocephalus depend on the age of onset. In early infancy, before closure of cranial sutures, head enlargement is the most common presentation, but in older children with less elasticity in the skull, neurological symptoms usually relate to increasing pressure on structures of the brain:

- *Early infancy:* bulging, non-pulsating fontanels (usually anterior) usually with increasing head circumference, dilated scalp veins, separating sutures, and positive Macewen sign (resonance on tapping near the frontal-temporal-parietal juncture).
- *Later signs:* enlargement of frontal area with depressed eyes, setting sun sign (sclera evident above iris), and pupils sluggish and unequally reactive.
- *Throughout infancy:* Increased irritability, lethargy, high-pitched crying, delayed responses, change in level of consciousness, opisthotonos, spasticity, difficulty feeding, and cardiopulmonary compromise.
- *Childhood* (related to increased intracranial pressure): Headache relieved by vomiting, papilledema, strabismus, ataxia, irritability, lethargy, confusion, and difficulty communicating.

Treatment

Hydrocephalus is diagnosed through CT and MRI, which help to determine the cause. Treatment may vary somewhat depending upon the underlying disorder, which may require treatment. For example, if obstruction is caused by a tumor, surgical excision to directly remove the obstruction is required. Generally, however, most hydrocephalus is **treated** with shunts:

- *Ventricular-peritoneal shunt:* This procedure is the most common and consists of placement of a ventricular catheter directly into the ventricles (usually lateral) at one end with the other end in the peritoneal area to drain away excess CSF. There is a one-way valve near the proximal end that prevents backflow but opens when pressure rises to drain fluid. In some cases, the distal end drains into the right atrium.
- *Third ventriculostomy:* A small opening is made in the base of the third ventricle so CSF can bypass an obstruction. This procedure is not common and is done with a small endoscope.

Bacterial Meningitis

Bacterial meningitis may be caused by a wide range of pathogenic organisms, with the predominant agents varying with the child's age:

- ≤1 month; E. coli, Group B streptococci, Listeria monocytogenes, and Neisseria meningitidis.
- 1-2 months: Group B streptococci.
- >2 months: Streptococcus pneumoniae, Neisseria meningitidis. Unvaccinated (Hib vaccine) children are at risk for Haemophilus influenzae.

Bacterial infections usually arise from spread distant infections although they can enter the CNS from surgical wounds, invasive devices, nasal colonization, or penetrating trauma. The infective process includes inflammation, exudates, white blood cell accumulation, and tissue damage with the brain showing evidence of hyperemia and edema. Purulent exudate covers the brain and invades and blocks the ventricles, obstructing CSF and leading to increased intracranial pressure. Since antibodies specific to bacteria don't cross the blood/brain barrier, the body's ability to fight the infection is very poor. Diagnosis is usually based on lumbar puncture examination of cerebrospinal fluid and symptoms.

Age-Related Symptoms

Bacterial meningitis may manifest differently, depending upon the age of the child:

- *Neonates*: Signs may be very non-specific, such as weight loss, hypo- or hyperthermia, jaundice, irritability, lethargy, irregular respirations with periods of apnea. More specific signs may include increasing signs of illness, difficulty feeding with loss of suck reflex, hypotonia, weak cry, seizures, and bulging fontanels (may be a late sign). Nuchal rigidity does not usually occur with neonates.
- *Infants and young children*: Classic symptoms usually don't appear until ≥2 years. Signs may include fever, poor feeding, vomiting, irritability, and bulging fontanel. Nuchal rigidity in some children.
- *Older children and adolescents:* Abrupt onset, including fever, chills, headache, and alterations of consciousness with seizures, agitation, and irritability. May have photophobia, hallucinations, aggressive behavior or stuporous and lapsing into coma. Nuchal rigidity progressing to opisthotonos. Reflexes are variable but positive Kernig and Brudzinski signs. Signs may relate to particular bacteria, such as rashes, sore joints, or draining ear.

Infectious Encephalopathy

Infectious encephalopathy is an encompassing term describing encephalopathies caused by a wide range of bacteria, viruses, or prions. Common to all infections are altered brain function that results in alterations in consciousness and personality, cognitive impairment, and lethargy. A wide range of neurological symptoms may occur: myoclonus, seizures, dysphagia, and dysphonia, neuromuscular impairment with muscle atrophy and tremors or spasticity. Treatment depends on the underlying cause and response to treatment. Prior infections are not treatable, but bacterial infections may respond to antibiotic therapy and viral infections may be self-limiting. HIV-related encephalopathy results from opportunistic infections as immune responses decrease, usually indicated by CD4 counts <50. Aggressive antiretroviral treatment and treatment of the infection may reverse symptoms if permanent damage has not occurred for HIV-related encephalopathy. Treatment for other infectious encephalopathies varies according to the type of infection and underlying causes.

Congenital Infections Related to Neurological Disease

Varicella Zoster Virus (Chicken Pox)

Chicken pox, caused by the **varicella zoster virus,** during the first 20 weeks of pregnancy can result in as infant with congenital varicella syndrome, which can cause a number of abnormalities of the skin, extremities, eyes, and central nervous system. Children are often unusually small with distinctive cicatrix scarring on the skin, and chorioretinitis. Brain abnormalities may include microcephaly, hydrocephalus, cortical atrophy, enlargement of the ventricles, and damage to the sympathetic nervous system. The child may suffer intellectual disability and developmental delays as well as lack of psychomotor coordination. If the mother is infected at the end of pregnancy and develops a rash from 5 days before to 2 days after delivery, the child may develop neonatal varicella, which poses of high risk to the child with mortality rates of about 30%. Vaccination prior to pregnancy is the best preventive. Premature neonates exposed after birth with ≤28 weeks gestation or ≥28 weeks if mother has no immunity should receive varicella zoster immunoglobulin (VZIG).

Toxoplasma Gondii

Toxoplasma gondii, is a single-celled parasite that transmitted from cat feces, poorly-cooked or raw meat, and if a pregnant woman is infected with toxoplasmosis, the infant can develop congenital toxoplasmosis, with transmission rates estimated at 20-50%. Symptoms in the neonate are most severe if the mother developed the infection in the first trimester. Congenital abnormalities include hydrocephalus, cerebral calcifications, chorioretinitis (classic triad of disorders). Additionally, the child may suffer from seizure disorders, microcephaly, and encephalitis. There may be other abnormalities as well, including hepatomegaly, splenomegaly, anemia, jaundice, and deafness. Treatment of the infected mother to prevent transmission to the fetus includes initially spiramycin (Rovamycin®), which reduces risk. Pyrimethamine (Daraprim®) and sulfonamide are usually given after the 18th week. Some studies have indicated that treatment does not reduce the rate of mother-infant transmission but does reduce the severity of abnormalities that child manifests.

Rubella and Cytomegalovirus

Rubella virus is an RNA virus that causes rubella (German measles), but infection in a pregnant woman during the first or second trimester can transmit to the infant congenital rubella syndrome (CRS), which can result in eye defects, congenital heart defects, hearing loss, hepatomegaly and hyperbilirubinemia and a number of defects of the central nervous system: microencephaly, seizures, and intellectual disability, delay in development, and meningoencephalitis. With vaccinations, this condition is now extremely rare in the United States.

Cytomegalovirus (CMV) infection during pregnancy can transmit to the infant cytomegalic inclusion disease, which can cause respiratory infections, bleeding, anemia, hepatic disorders, and vision impairment. Central nervous system defects include microcephaly, cerebral calcifications, seizure disorders and intellectual disability. CMV is the virus most frequently transmitted congenitally and most infants suffer no ill effects, but some develop severe disabilities. Infants of mothers with their first infection during pregnancy are at highest risk for developing abnormalities.

Neurologic Infectious Diseases

West Nile Virus

West Nile Virus is an RNA virus, spread by infected mosquitoes. Infection has been traced to donor organs, blood transfusions, and breast milk although the blood supply has been monitored for WNV since 2003. While WNV is more common in adult, especially the elderly, it can affect infants and children. Infected children show symptoms more readily than adults. The incubation period ranges from 2-14 days. There are 3 types of infection:

- *Viremia*: 80%, infection but no symptoms.
- *Mild*: 20% (West Nile fever), characterized by fever, malaise, lymphadenopathy, headache, rash, nausea, and vomiting. The acute stage is usually is self-limiting within a few days, but symptoms can persist for weeks, including muscular weakness, fatigue, concentration problems, fever, and headache. About 30% require hospitalization.
- *Severe*: <1%, severe neurological symptoms with meningitis and associated symptoms being the most common in children and young adults.

Treatment is supportive during illness and preventive (insect repellant).

Arboviruses

There are a number of **arboviruses** in addition to West Nile Virus that can cause flu-like symptoms that progress to viral encephalitis, and incidence is increasing across the United States, often spread by mosquitoes. Because many people are unaware of emerging causes for diseases, the cause of the ensuing encephalitis is frequently misdiagnosed. Encephalitis is an infection of the brain tissue and usually lasts for 2-3 weeks. **Symptoms** vary somewhat from one type of infection to another, but they have similar characteristics.

- Onset usually involves flu-like symptoms with sore throat, headaches, muscle aches, fever and chills, myalgia. In some cases, a rash may appear.
- Progressive symptoms include photophobia, vomiting, and increased weakness.
- Advanced symptoms may include altered mental status, seizures, memory loss, coma, and death.

Encephalitis may also result from complications of Lyme disease, spread by infected ticks. One of the most common causes of encephalitis is the herpes simplex virus.

Arboviral Encephalitides Found in the U.S.
Arboviral encephalitides include:

- *Eastern equine encephalitis virus (EEEV)* (Togaviridae) has a high mortality rate and is most common in the eastern and gulf coast areas of the U.S. Sporadic outbreaks occur. Half of survivors have residual neurological damage, especially children.
- *Western equine encephalitis (WEE)* (Togaviridae) is similar to EEE but found on the west coast and the Midwest.
- Venezuelan equine encephalitis (Togaviridae) occurs primarily in Florida and southwest U.S.
- *St. Louis encephalitis* (Flaviviridae) occurs throughout the U.S. but most infections are sub-clinical; however, if symptoms are present, about 50% of those under age 20 develop encephalitis and 5-15% die.
- *La Cross encephalitis* (Bunyaviridae) is scattered and rare and usually results in mild disease with mortality rate <1%.
- *Cache Valley virus* (Bunyaviridae) has occurred in southeast and Wisconsin and is believed to be under-reported. It occurs primarily in children <16. Mortality rates are <1% but neurological damage may persist.

Seizure Disorders

Seizures are sudden involuntary abnormal electrical disturbances in the brain that can manifest as alterations of consciousness, spastic tonic and clonic movements, convulsions, and loss of consciousness. Seizures are a symptom of underlying pathology. Many seizures are transient, such as febrile seizures in children ≤2 years old. Some seizures may result from pathology, such as meningitis, cerebral edema, brain trauma, or brain tumors, but most seizures in children >3 are related to idiopathic epilepsy, which predisposes the child to recurrent seizures, usually of the same type. Seizures are believed caused by cells known as epileptogenic focus, which increase electrical discharge in response to physiological changes, such as fatigue or changes in blood sugar level. The electrical discharge spreads to the brainstem, causing generalized seizures. Seizures are characterized as focal (localized), focal with rapid generalization (spreading) and generalized (widespread). In most children, seizures become generalized with loss of consciousness. Seizure disorders with onset <4 usually cause more neurological damage than those >4.

Partial Seizures

Partial seizures are caused by an electrical discharged to a localized area of the cerebral cortex, such as the frontals, temporal, or parietal lobes with seizure characteristics related to area of involvement. They may begin in a focal area and become generalized, often preceded by an aura.

- *Simple partial:* unilateral motor symptoms including somatosensory, psychic, and autonomic.
- *Aversive:* eyes and head turned away from focal side.
- *Sylvan* (usually during sleep): tonic-clonic movements of the face, salivation, and arrested speech.
- *Special sensory:* various sensations (numbness, tingling, prickling, or pain) spreading from one area. May include visual sensations, posturing or hypertonia. Rare <8 years.
- *Complex (Psychomotor):* No loss of consciousness, but altered consciousness and non-responsive with amnesia. May involve complex sensorium with bad tastes, auditory or visual hallucinations, feeling of déjà vu, strong fear. May carry out repetitive activities, such as walking, running, smacking lips, chewing, or drawling. Rarely aggressive. Seizure usually followed by prolonged drowsiness and confusion. Occurs 3 through adolescence.

Generalized Seizures

Generalized seizures lack a focal onset and appear to involve both hemispheres, usually presenting with loss of consciousness and no preceding aura.

- Tonic-clonic (Grand Mal): Occurs without warning.
  - Tonic period (10-30 seconds): Eyes roll upward with loss of consciousness, arms flexed, stiffen in symmetric tonic contraction of body, apneic with cyanosis and salivating.
  - Clonic period (10 seconds to 30 minutes, but usually 30 seconds). Violent rhythmic jerking with contraction and relaxation. May be incontinent of urine and feces. Contractions slow and then stop.
- Following seizures, there may be confusion, disorientation, impairment of motor activity, speech and vision for several hours. May involve headache, nausea, and vomiting. Child often falls asleep and awakens conscious.
- *Absence (Petit Mal):* Onset between 4-12 and usually ends in puberty. Onset is abrupt with brief loss of consciousness for 5-10 seconds and slight loss of muscle tone but often appears to be daydreaming. May include lip smacking or eye twitching.

- *Atonic and akinetic (drop attacks):* Onset 2-5 years. Sudden loss of muscle tone and control of posture causes child to fall violently to the floor. Loss of consciousness may be momentary. May recur frequently during the daytime, and child may have serious injuries from falls.
- *Myoclonic seizures:* Sudden brief muscle contractures, single or repetitively. May be symmetric. No loss of consciousness, and may occur independently or associated with other types of seizures.
- *Infantile myoclonus (spasm):* Occurs ≤ 8 months, more commonly in males. Series of sudden short, symmetric muscle contractions with head flexed, arms extended, and knees drawn up OR extensor spasms of trunk and head nodding. May occur repeatedly during day. May have "lightning" very short momentary contraction of body. May lose consciousness and eyes may roll upward. Often causes cognitive impairment.

Status Epilepticus

Status epilepticus (SE) is usually generalized tonic-clonic seizures that are characterized by a series of seizures with intervening time too short for regaining of consciousness. The constant assault and periods of apnea can lead to exhaustion, respiratory failure with hypoxemia and hypercapnia, cardiac failure, and death. There are a number of causes of SE:

- Uncontrolled epilepsy or non-compliance with anticonvulsants.
- Infections, such as encephalitis.
- Encephalopathy or brain attack.
- Drug toxicity (isoniazid).
- Brain trauma.
- Neoplasms.
- Metabolic disorders.

Treatment includes:

Anticonvulsants, usually beginnings with fast-acting benzodiazepine (Ativan®), often in steps, with administration of medication every 5 minutes until seizures subside. If cause is undetermined, acyclovir and ceftriaxone may be administered. If there is no response to the first 2 doses of anticonvulsants (refractory SE), rapid sequence intubation (RSI), which involves sedation and paralytic anesthesia may be done while therapy continues. Combining phenobarbital and benzodiazepine can cause apnea, so intubation may be necessary. Phenytoin and phenobarbital are added.

Brain Tumors in Infants and Children

Any type of **brain tumor** can occur in children, but the most common are those that arise from immature (blast) cells or supportive (glial) tissue. The most common age group for children with brain tumors is 3-12.

- *Astrocytoma:* This arises from astrocytes, which are glial cells. It is the most common type of tumor. It can occur throughout the brain but is most common in the cerebellum of children. There are many types of astrocytomas, and most are slow growing. Some are operable; others are not. Radiation may be given after removal.
- *Brain stem glioma:* This may be fast or slow growing but is generally not operable because of location although it may be treated with radiation or chemotherapy.

- *Craniopharyngioma:* This is a congenital, slow-growing, and benign cystic tumor but difficult to resect, and treated with surgery and radiation. They may be recurrent, especially if >5cm so early excision is important.
- *Ependymoma:* This is usually benign in a cerebral hemisphere. Surgical excision and radiation are done.
- *Ganglioglioma:* This can occur anywhere in the brain but 70% in children occur above the tentorium (the membrane separating the cerebellum from the occipital lobes. They are usually slow growing and benign. *Medulloblastoma:* There are many types of medulloblastoma, most arising in the cerebellum, malignant, and fast growing. Surgical excision is done and often followed by radiation and chemotherapy although recent studies show using just chemotherapy controls recurrence with less neurological damage.
- *Oligodendroglioma:* This tumor most often occurs in the cerebrum, primarily the frontal or temporal lobes, involving the myelin sheath of the neurons.
- *Optical nerve glioma:* This slow growing tumor of the optic nerve is usually a form of astrocytoma. It is often associated with neurofibromatosis type I (NF1), occurring in 15-40%. Despite surgical, chemotherapy or radiotherapy treatment, it is usually fatal.

Cerebral Palsy

Cerebral palsy (CP) is a non-progressive motor dysfunction related to CNS damage associated with congenital, hypoxic, or traumatic injury before, during, or ≤2 years after birth. It may include visual defects, speech impairment, seizures and intellectual disability. There are 4 types of motor dysfunction:

- *Spastic*: Damage to the cerebral cortex or pyramidal tract. Constant hypertonia and rigidity lead to contractures and curvature of the spine.
- *Dyskinetic*: Damage to the extrapyramidal, basal ganglia. Tremors and twisting with exaggerated posturing and impairment of voluntary muscle control.
- *Ataxic*: Damage to the extrapyramidal cerebellum. Atonic muscles in infancy with lack of balance, instability of muscles and poor gait.
- *Mixed*: Combinations of all three types with multiple areas of damage.

Characteristics of CP include:

- Hypotonia or hypertonia with rigidity and spasticity.
- Athetosis (constant writhing motions)
- Ataxia
- Hemiplegia (one-sided involvement, more severe in upper extremities)
- Diplegia (all extremities involved, but more severe in lower extremities)
- Quadriplegia (all extremities involved with arms flexed and legs extended)

Management

Cerebral palsy requires a multidisciplinary approach to treatment, depending upon the type and extent of impairment. CP may not be detected for 4-6 months or even longer after birth when developmental delays or spastic movements become apparent.

- Visual deficits, such as strabismus, may require repair.
- Hearing loss may interfere with language acquisition.
- Speech therapy is often needed.
- Physical and occupational therapy to help maximize potential.

- Bowel and bladder training may not be complete until 3-10 years.
- Special education to help the child in school.
- Surgical repairs are often multiple:
  - Lengthening of Achilles' tendon to improve gait.
  - Release of hamstrings to reverse flexion contractures of knees.
  - Repair of hips to improve abduction.
  - Foot surgery to correct position of foot for ambulation.

Some children will remain dependent on others and require lifetime assistance with activities of daily living, but others will be able to function independently.

Review of Systems: Musculoskeletal

Genu Varum and Genu Valgum

Genu varum (bowlegs) and **genu valgum (knock-kneed)** are normal progressions in straightening of the legs. Genu varum (lateral bowing of the tibia) is present in infants until after they begin to walk and strengthen muscles. It is clinically significant if the measured distance between the knees is >2 inches (5 cm) or if it persists beyond age 2-3. As the legs begin to straighten the next stage is genu valgum in which the knees come together with the ankles separated. Children remain knock-kneed from about ages 2-5 although it may persist until age 7 in some children. It is clinically significant if the measured distance between the ankles (malleoli) is >3 inches (7.5 cm) or if it persists after about age 7, at which time the legs should straighten so the child can stand with the knees and ankles together.

Legg-Calvé-Perthes Disease

Legg-Calvé-Perthes disease is avascular necrosis of the femoral head resulting from compromised blood supply, which may result from genetic predisposition, traumatic injury, low birth weight, and exposure to environmental tobacco smoke. It is most common between 2-12 with peak incidence at 4-8, affecting boys 4 times more than girls. There are 5 stages:

- Pre-necrotic injury interferes with blood supply.
- Necrosis (3-6 months) is the avascular stage with mild pain or limp but normal radiograph.
- Revascularization (1l-4 years) with pain and limited movement and sometimes fractures of the femoral head. Necrotic bone is resorbed and new bone deposited.
- Healing involves reossification of bone and decrease in pain.
- Remodeling is the end of the healing process with no pain and improved function.

Treatment to prevent pain and deformity;

- Traction to maintain abduction followed by Petrie (abduction) casting

OR

- Adductor tenotomy followed by Toronto (abduction) brace.

DDH

Developmental displacement of the hip (DDH) comprises disorders in which the femoral head and the acetabulum are misaligned:

- *Dislocation*: The femoral head displaced from the joint.
- *Subluxation*: The hip unstable, and the femoral head slides in and out of the joint.
- *Dysplasia*: Structural joint abnormality with a shallow acetabulum.

About 1% of infants have some hip instability at birth, but more serious disorders are less common, affecting 4 times more girls than boys with 80% unilateral, and the left side affected 3 times more than the right. **Causes** include:

- Genetic component.
- Maternal estrogen may cause laxity of the joint.
- Breech birth may cause traumatic injury.
- Cultural factors, such as swaddling infant with legs extended.
- Injury.

Diagnosis is with ultrasound in neonates and x-rays after 2-3 months. Children have limited abduction with asymmetry of fat folds. Older children limp. **Treatment**:

- Pavlik harness to maintain flexed, abducted position.
- Open reduction and cast may be needed in severe cases.

Osteogenesis Imperfecta

Osteogenesis imperfecta (OI) is a genetic disorder (usually autosomal dominant), which results in a biochemical defect in the production of collagen, affecting connective tissue and resulting in fragile bones ("brittle bone disease"). OI is characterized by frequent and multiple fractures, blue sclerae, thin soft skin, ↑ joint flexibility, enlarged anterior fontanel, weak muscles, dentinogenesis imperfecta (weak dentin and discolored teeth), and short stature. There are currently 7 classifications:

1. This is the mildest and most common form. Blue sclerae occurs but teeth are often normal. Fractures usually occur when the child begins to walk and cease after puberty. The child usually attains normal stature.
2. This is the most severe form with the child born with multiple fractures and surviving only a few days.
3. This is the most severe form that allows survival, but infant is often born with fractures and incurs multiple fractures through childhood, continuing to adulthood, resulting in very short stature. Most are confined to wheelchairs.
4. This is a varied form with some having multiple fractures and deformities with short stature and others a less severe form with more normal stature.
5. This form causes moderate to severe deformities with a range of bone fragility but without blue sclerae or dentinogenesis imperfecta. There is hypertrophic callus formation.
6. Similar to type V but osteoid accumulates in bones resulting in osteomalacia.
7. Similar to type V but with shortening of the humerus and femur. This form is autosomal recessive.

123

There is no cure for OI, so **management goals** are to prevent fractures and deformity and control pain:

- Physical therapy.
- Casting.
- Braces or splints.
- Surgical repair.
- High vitamin D and calcium in diet.
- Bisphosphonate medications (pamidronate) IV every 4-6 months has been shown to reduce bone fractures and pain.
- Bone marrow transplant has been successful with some cases of severe OI.

Spinal Fusion for Children and Adolescents

Spinal fusion is done to repair vertebral abnormalities, some resulting in spinal curvature of the spine with disability and deformity that can impair cardiopulmonary function and cause death. While exercises, braces, and electrical stimulation are used to treat mild conditions, surgical correction is often required:

- Spinal fusion usually includes spinal realignment and straightening with vertebrae fused together with bone grafts, usually from the child's iliac crest or a donor.
- The grafts may be placed posteriorly or anteriorly, often with the addition of instrumentation (hardware) in the form of rods, screws, wires, hooks, plates, and cages to stabilize and align vertebrae during fusion.
- A posterior fusion is done with a vertical incision along the length of the spine to be fused.
- An anterior fusion requires an incision will be back to front on one side of the rib cage (thoracic repair) or across rib cage and down the abdomen (for thoracic and lumbar repair).
- Endoscopic surgery may be done through small incisions.

Musculoskeletal Conditions That May Require Spinal Fusion for Correction

Spinal fusion may be needed for the following conditions:

- *Kyphosis*, a convex angulation of the thoracic spine, may be secondary, such as to arthritis or compression fractures, or may be postural, resulting from skeletal growth faster than muscular. Exercises may help postural kyphosis.
- *Lordosis,* an often-painful concave angulation of the lumbar spine, frequently associated with obesity, flexion hip contracture, and slipped femoral capital epiphysis. Exercises may give some relief but not a permanent cure.
- *Scoliosis*, a lateral and rotational curvature of the spine, can cause alterations in the structure of the pelvis and chest. It may be nonstructural, related to some other deformity or underlying problem, or structural, with changes in the spine and vertebrae because of congenital or other disorders. It is idiopathic in 70-80% of cases.
- *Spina bifida*, a neural tube defect, results in incomplete closure of the spine with the bones over the defect underdeveloped and unfused.

A child may have a combination, such as scoliokyphosis.

Muscular Dystrophies

<u>Pseudohypertrophic (Duchenne)</u>

Pseudohypertrophic (Duchenne) muscular dystrophy is the most common form and the most severe. It is an X-linked disorder in about 50% of the cases with the rest sporadic mutations, affecting males almost exclusively. Children typically have some delay in motor development, with difficulty walking and have evidence of muscle weakness by about age 3. Pseudohypertrophic refers to enlargement of muscles by fatty infiltration associated with muscular atrophy, which causes contractures and deformities of joints. Abnormal bone development results in spinal and other skeletal deformities. The disease progresses rapidly, and most children are wheelchair bound by about 12 years of age. As the disease progresses, it involves the muscles of the diaphragm and other muscles needed for respiration. Mild to frank mental deficiency is common. Facial, oropharyngeal, and respiratory muscles weaken late in the disease. Cardiomegaly commonly occurs. Death most often relates to respiratory infection or cardiac failure by age 25. Treatment is supportive.

<u>Facioscapulohumeral Muscular Dystrophy and Limb-Girdle Muscular Dystrophy</u>

Muscular dystrophies are genetic disorders with gradual degeneration of muscle fibers and progressive weakness and atrophy of skeletal muscles and loss of mobility. Types differ according to the muscles involved, the age of onset, and the speed of progression:

- *Facioscapulohumeral muscular dystrophy* (Landouzy-Dejerine) is a slowly-progressive autosomal recessive disorder with onset usually between 10-24. Typically, the shoulder angle forward, the face loses mobility, and the child cannot raise the arms above the head because of weakness of the upper arms. The lower extremities may be affected as the disease progresses.
- *Limb-girdle muscular dystrophy* is a group of autosomal recessive or dominant disorders with onset in later childhood or adolescence, manifesting as weakness of proximal muscles of the pelvic and shoulder girdles although muscles in proximity to these (upper arms and thighs) may weaken over time. There are over a dozen forms, related to specific genetic defects. Some forms cause serious disability in a few years and others progress very slowly.

Progressive Infantile Muscular Atrophy

Progressive infantile muscular atrophy (Werdnig-Hoffman disease) is am autosomal recessive inherited disorder ("floppy infant syndrome") with progressive weakness and wasting of skeletal muscles caused by degeneration of anterior horn cells of the spinal cord and the motor nuclei of the brainstem. There are 3 different groups of the disorder, characterized by different onset and symptoms:

- *Group I:* Most severe with onset ≤2 months. Children are alert with normal intellect but weak and inactive and have little movement of extremities except for fingers and toes. The motor skills do not progress and the child usually dies by age 3.
- *Group 2:* Onset is 2-12 months and progresses from weakness of arms and legs to generalized. Pectus excavatum is prominent. Life expectancy ranges from 7 months to 7 years.
- *Group 3:* Onset in 2nd year with normal control of head but thigh and hip muscles weak and there is lumbar lordosis, waddling gait and protruding abdomen. Child is usually wheelchair bound between 10-20.

Review of Systems: Immune System

Management of Bacterial Infections

Erysipelas

Erysipelas is a superficial bacterial infection, primarily of the face or legs, involving the cutaneous lymphatic system and invading the skin in areas of trauma. Facial erysipelas is usually caused by group A *Streptococcus* following a nasopharyngeal infection. Infections on the legs are more often related to non-group A *Streptococcus*. The infection spreads rapidly with streaking and clearly demarcated erythema and cellulitis. Local lymph nodes become inflamed, sometimes resulting in lymphedema because of damage to lymph nodes. Erysipelas most commonly affects children and the elderly. **Treatment** includes:

- Bed rest with elevation of affected limb and warm saline packs to improve circulation.
- Oral antibiotic (usually penicillin G and penicillin VK). IV antibiotics may be indicated for severe cases.
- Hospitalization is recommended for severe cases or those who are very young, elderly, or immunocompromised.
- Analgesics to control pain.

MRSA

Methicillin-resistant *Staphylococcus aureus* (MRSA) is caused by a mutation in *S. aureus*, causing it to be resistant to methicillin (amoxicillin) and other beta lactamase-resistant penicillins as well as cephalosporins. First identified in 1945, MRSA has become endemic in hospitals and is increasingly the cause of surgical site and bloodstream infections and pneumonia with over half of *S. aureus* infections now MRSA and mortality rates of 21%. MRSA infection rates in children have risen sharply. MRSA is often colonized on the skin, especially in the anterior nares, and can easily spread through contact with contaminated surfaces or hands. Community-acquired MRSA is also increasing, especially among children, and can precipitate sepsis and a severe necrotizing pneumonia:

Treatment includes the following:

- Prompt diagnosis and treatment with Vancomycin or other antibiotics.
- Standard and contact precautions with use of gloves, gown, and masks with pneumonia.
- Droplet precautions with pneumonia.

Place child in private room or cohort.

SSSS

***Staphylococcal* scalded skin syndrome (SSSS)** is a superficial partial-thickness infection of the skin caused by toxins produced by a localized *Staphylococcus aureus* infection, resulting in generalized erythema followed in 24-48 hours with blisters that rupture and peel off, leaving large areas of superficial necrosis and denuded skin, giving the skin a burned or "scalded" appearance. It is most common in neonates and children under 5 but can affect adults who are immunocompromised or in renal failure. Pain is usually mild unless the infection is very widespread. **Treatment** includes:

- IV antibiotics (such as flucloxacillin) are usually needed initially, followed by a course of oral antibiotics.
- Maintenance of fluids and electrolytes.
- Debridement of skin.
- Moisture-retentive dressings, such as foam dressings, sheet hydrogels, and alginates, avoiding adhesives.
- Excessive tissue loss may be treated the same as partial-thickness burns.

Management for Fungal Infections

Candidiasis

Candidiasis, infection of the epidermis with *Candida* spp. (commonly referred to as "yeast" or "thrush"), causes a pustular erythematous papular rash that is commonly scaly, crusty, and macerated with a white cheese-like exudate. It may burn and is usually extremely pruritic and grows in warm moist areas of the skin, such as under breasts and abdominal folds and the perineal area. Antibiotic use, immunocompromised status, and diabetes mellitus may predispose people to fungal infections, so candidiasis must be differentiated from bacterial infections because antibiotic treatment will worsen the condition. **Treatment** includes:

- Preventing humid moist conditions of skin.
- Controlling hyperglycemia.
- Burrows solutions soaks with air-drying to relieve itching.
- Topical antifungal creams (clotrimazole, nystatin, fluconazole, and ketoconazole) twice daily.
- Topical antifungal powders for mild cases.
- Oral antifungal medications for severe cases.

Tinea Cruris and Tinea Pedis

Tinea cruris (jock itch) is a fungal infection of the perineal area, penis, inner thighs, and inguinal creases, but may also occur under breasts in women and beneath abdominal folds where skin is warm and moist. It rarely occurs before adolescence. **Symptoms** include: Scaly, itching, erythematous rash that may contain papules or vesicle and is usually bilateral and symmetrical.

Treatment includes the following:

- Selenium sulfide shampoo wash of area before applying medication.
- Topical antifungal (clotrimazole, miconazole, tolnaftate, naftifine, terbinafine) 2 times daily for 4 weeks.

Tinea pedis (athlete's foot) is a fungal infection of the feet and toes. It is rare before adolescence and is more common in males. *Symptoms* include: Severe itching with vesicles or erosion of instep and with peeling maceration and fissures between toes. Dry scaly mildly erythematous patches on plantar and lateral foot surfaces.

Treatment includes the following:

- Same as tinea cruris.
- Keep feet dry with absorbent talc.
- Allow feet to air dry and use 100% cotton socks, change twice daily.

Tinea Capitis and Tinea Corporis

Tinea capitis is a fungal infection of the scalp, usually affecting children between 1-10. It is spread through the sharing of combs, brushes, or caps. **Symptoms** include: Circumscribed areas of hair loss with fine scaling and superficial pustules with mild itching.

Treatment includes the following:

- Griseofulvin orally 8-12 weeks.
- Selenium sulfide shampoo 2-3 times weekly, leaving shampoo on scalp for 10 minutes before rinsing.

Tinea corporis is a fungal infection of the skin of the trunk although it can occur on the face or other parts of the body, affecting both children and teenagers. It is spread by direct contact. **Symptoms** include:

One or multiple circular patches that may be scaly and erythematous with slightly raised borders.

Treatment includes the following:

- Selenium sulfide shampoo wash of area before applying medication.
- Topical antifungal (clotrimazole, miconazole, tolnaftate, naftifine, terbinafine) 2 times daily for 4 weeks.